Handbook and Atlas of Gastrointestinal Exfoliative Cytology

João Carlos Prolla and Joseph B. Kirsner

The University of Chicago Press

Chicago and London

The University of Chicago Press, Chicago 60637
The University of Chicago Press, Ltd., London

This book is dedicated to Maurice Goldblatt,

humanitarian, great benefactor, and longtime supporter of research in cancer

Contents

Preface

This book was written for two main purposes: to review our more than twenty years of personal experience with the clinical applications of gastrointestinal cytology and to prepare a guide for those interested in establishing this science in their laboratories.

Interest in gastrointestinal exfoliative cytology at the University of Chicago began in 1950 with Dr. Cyrus E. Rubin, now professor of medicine at the University of Washington in Seattle. He initiated the original techniques and established the clinical usefulness of the method, as well as stimulating a variety of research projects. Dr. Howard Raskin, now associate professor of medicine at the University of Maryland in Baltimore, introduced further technical modifications, including a rapid method for duodenal intubation, and also extended the diagnostic horizons of the gastrointestinal cytologic method in cancer diagnosis. Other physicians who have made useful contributions to this work at the University of Chicago include Dr. Melvin I. Klayman, now a staff member at the Beth Israel Hospital in Massachusetts; Dr. Kenneth Barton, assistant professor of medicine at the University of San Francisco and Dr. Duane Taebel, now at the Gundersen Clinic in Wisconsin. Their contributions illustrate the continuity so necessary in productive research and attest that progress often depends upon a succession of scientific developments rather than upon a single event.

To place our personal clinical experience with gastrointestinal cytology in proper perspective, we comprehensively reviewed the world's literature, seeking new methodologic approaches and promising research applications. The complete integration of endoscopy and cytology now appears to be the best approach to applying both procedures in the clinical examination of the esophagus, stomach, and duodeno-biliary-pancreatic areas of the gastrointestinal tract and later perhaps the colon and rectum. This advance should decrease the need for specialized laboratories exclusively for gastrointestinal cytology. These expensive units were almost indispensable two decades ago, when fluid washing methods were the only techniques available. And because of the difficulties of such procedures, only highly specialized units could achieve reasonably accurate results. However, the endoscopist with the responsibility of procuring adequate cytologic material should be wary lest the simplicity of the direct-vision techniques encourage careless techniques. Meticulous care always will be essential to successful gastrointestinal cytology. The future role of cytology in mass screening in countries with a high incidence of gastric carcinoma deserves careful study. We considered it appropriate to include one chapter on this and to suggest guidelines based upon present knowledge.

The second objective of this book is to help those beginning to study the technical and morphological details of gastrointestinal cytology. The chapters of the cell collection and processing and the staining of the exfoliated cellular material, as well as the iconographic chapters, were prepared with this in mind. The advanced reader may criticize the absence of histopathological illustrations, but, in our judgment, to include in-depth discussion of histopathological findings would confuse the technical staff reader without necessarily enhancing the value of this manual.

Certainly there is no substitute for direct personal study of cytological preparations under the guidance of an experienced cytologist. But we think that a collection of representative photomicrographs could be a useful complement. Chapters 14 and 15 describe our personal experience with gastrointestinal cytology and give the most important diagnostic criteria of gastrointestinal neoplasia.

Acknowledgments

This book would not have been possible without the cooperation and encouragement of many colleagues and the generous collaboration of our cytotechnicians. We are particularly grateful to Dr. Seibi Kobayashi and Dr. Rogerio G. Xavier. To Dr. Kobayashi we owe important assistance in the procedure of direct-vision cytology, and to Dr. Xavier, our experience with the Acridine-Orange and the Shorr staining techniques. The technical help of our staff of cytotechnicians was particularly important, and the high accuracy of our diagnostic cytology is due mainly to their skill and motivation. We are particularly grateful to Leroy Cockerham, who has been our chief cytotechnician since 1959.

The generous financial support of Maurice Goldblatt, whose lifelong interest in cancer research and concern for humanity have led him to support and stimulate the development of this book, is gratefully acknowledged.

Dr. Prolla received a fellowship from the Gastro-Intestinal Research Foundation during the period when the book was written, and was granted a leave of absence from his original institution (Pôrto Alegre Medical School, Federal University of Rio Grande do Sul, Pôrto Alegre, Brazil). The generous support of these two groups is gratefully acknowledged. Finally, we wish to extend our appreciation to our secretarial staff, whose skillful retypings aided immensely in the development of the final text.

1

Introduction

Since the pioneer work of Papanicolaou and his collaborators, the modern application of exfoliative cytology—or diagnostic cytology, the term preferred by L. G. Koss—has developed along two main lines. The first is its use as a clinical diagnostic tool for patients with symptoms of diseases of various organs and systems. Its second use is as a mass survey tool to discover unsuspected malignant tumors in apparently asymptomatic populations. It has been used especially to detect uterine cervical cancer and, to a much lesser extent, to screen asymptomatic smokers for bronchogenic carcinoma by sputum cytology and for oral cancer by oral cytology.

The clinical application of gastrointestinal cytology in evaluating patients with symptoms of disease of the gastrointestinal tract is well documented. But we would like to emphasize its role in cancer detection and to caution against attempting to use it to diagnose other pathological processes. The specificity of the findings is too low to make them of practical value for this, and wide use of the method under such circumstances could cause it to be unjustifiably discredited.

Developments in fiber endoscopy have been especially important and have facilitated the development of the "direct-vision" approach. The exact source of the cells can now be determined, and the sampling error in the collection of the material is being decreased by an extremely simple procedure. We hope that the development of safe and practical duodenoscopes and colonoscopes, which has already been reported, will bring patients with duodenal and colonic lesions the same diagnostic benefits that the fiber-esophagoscopes and fiber-gastroscopes have brought to those with diseases of the esophagus and the stomach.

In the clinical context, radiology, endoscopy, and cytology are complementary, and comparisons of "diagnostic accuracy" are misleading and may be biased. Radiology preferably should be undertaken first. Then endoscopy may help decide the nature of any lesion detected, discover lesions not visible by radiology, or rule out suspected lesions. The endoscopist usually benefits greatly from the roentgen studies of the patient, and this information should be utilized both in planning the examination and in evaluating the lesion.

Diagnostic cytology will further clarify the radiologic-endoscopic diagnosis and accurately characterize malignant tumors in many areas of the gastrointestinal tract. A negative diagnostic cytology report should not be overemphasized, however, and should be used only as circumstantial evidence of the absence of a malignant process. The direct-vision method will facilitate the use of these three basic diagnostic methods, because cytology is performed at the same time as endoscopy. This saves the time of the patient (reducing hospitalization costs) and of the medical and paramedical personnel (always at premium), and decreases the sampling error to almost zero (148).

Meticulous technical care is most important in all the cytological procedures described and cannot be overemphasized. This principle is much more important than selecting a staining method or even a cell collection method. As is described in detail in part 3, we have found that the sensitivity (or detection rate) of the cytological method is highest in gastroesophageal malignant tumors, where it approaches 90% by the direct-vision method. Malignant tumors of the colon occupy an intermediate position, with a detection rate of approximately 75%, and pancreatobiliary tumors are identified in slightly more than 50% of instances (table 1.1). In our experience, the specificity of the positive cytodiagnosis is remarkably similar in all areas; for approximately 95% of all positive reports the presence of malignant tumors is proved, and less than 5% of reports are "false positives" in the three main gastrointestinal areas under

TABLE 1.1

DETECTION RATE (SENSITIVITY) OF DIAGNOSTIC CYTOLOGY FOR PROVED MALIGNANT TUMORS OF THE GASTROINTESTINAL TRACT

Tumor Site	No. of Patients	Positive Cytology	Detection Rate (%)	Comments
Esophagus				
a) washing cytology	87	79	90.8	Includes some tumors of the cardia
b) direct-vision cytology	9	9	100.0	Only squamous cell carcinomas
Stomach				
a) washing cytology	379	288	76.6	. . .
b) direct-vision cytology	40	35	87.5	. . .
Duodenum, Pancreas, and Biliary Tract	182	107	58.7	. . .
Colon	112	87	77.6	Lesions beyond reach of sigmoidoscope

NOTE: University of Chicago series.

study (gastroesophageal, pancreatobiliary, and colonic) (table 1.2).

A somewhat different problem exists when mass surveys for upper gastrointestinal carcinomas are considered in countries with high incidence rates (such as Japan, Chile, or Germany). The main purpose of cytology, then, is to select patients for tissue examination at a minimum cost in money and in time of medical per-

TABLE 1.2

SPECIFICITY OF THE POSITIVE REPORT IN
GASTROINTESTINAL TRACT DIAGNOSTIC CYTOLOGY

Area under Study	No. of Positive Reports [a] (A)	Proved Malignant Tumors (B)	Ratio B/A × 100 (% Specificity)
Esophagus (washing cytology)	83	79	95.7
Stomach (washing cytology)	293	288	98.2
Esophagus and stomach (direct-vision cytology)	47	44	93.6
Duodenum, pancreas, and biliary tract	112	107	95.5
Colon	91	87	95.6

NOTE: University of Chicago series.
[a] Patients in whom a malignant tumor was found in a neighboring organ are not included here. The problem in such instances is to determine the origin of the cells and not the specificity of the positive report.

sonnel. Cytology fulfills its case-finding role adequately if it singles out for detailed clinical examinations or biopsy almost all gastric malignancies of a large asymptomatic population and produces a minimum of false-positives. The method should be simple, easy to perform, and reasonably well tolerated by most people. At present, lavage with saline solution, with or without alphachymotrypsin added, most closely approximates these requirements. The potential value of quick-staining procedures such as the use of Acridine Orange (fluorescence microscopy) and Shorr's polychromic method also should be recognized. In most countries, however, the use of exfoliative cytology in screening large unselected groups remains impractical because of the time required, the lack of trained personnel, and, in the United States, the relatively low incidence of gastric carcinoma. Gastrocamera examinations may be as useful as cytology, provided no effort is made to reach people with benign-appearing conditions. As we will explain in

chapter 9, a study comparing exfoliative cytology and gastrocamera is desirable to assure the proper emphasis. For malignancies of the duodenum, pancreas, and biliary tree there is no easy solution, but the immunological screening test for carcinoma of the pancreas proposed by Weiland, Kuntz, and Childers (289) may be interesting if it is confirmed in larger series. For carcinoma of the colon and rectum, periodic proctoscopic examination is the best approach, but a good screening method is still needed for carcinomas of the colon that are beyond reach of the proctoscope. Again, the immunological approach proposed by Gold and his colleagues (90, 278) may be helpful, although the technological problems are considerable. The use of longer flexible fibercolonoscopes also seems promising, if the technique can be improved to permit more rapid passage of the instrument.

The special problem of photofluorographic mass surveys for gastric carcinoma is discussed in chapter 9. The excessive number of false-positives or suspicious cases probably makes the cost per patient prohibitive, and the possible genetic hazard of radiation needs to be excluded completely.

The shortage of highly motivated and well-trained cytotechnologists is a barrier to more extensive use of exfoliative cytology in the diagnosis of gastrointestinal tumors. Their contribution is crucial in all cell-collection methods except the direct-vision technique. However, their role in screening the smears is less specialized, and cytotechnologists with adequate training in accredited schools can perform the screening well after a few weeks of special tutoring. The same is true for the cytopathologist; gastrointestinal cytology is no more difficult than other areas. The most difficult and most important step is adequate cell collection, which further emphasizes the importance of the new developments in endoscopy.

This book deals particularly with the use of diagnostic cytology in the management of patients with symptoms referable to the digestive tract. In part 2 we review the methodology used in our laboratory and elsewhere. Part 3 deals with our material and results, and includes a review of the pertinent literature. Part 4 describes cell morphology and is directed especially to cytologists and cytotechnicians interested in the morphological aspects of the subject. We have tried to include most of the cytological pictures likely to be encountered in the clinical applications of gastrointestinal cytology, and they are illustrated by appropriate photomicrographs.

2
Historical Notes

More than one hundred years ago, in the last half of the nineteenth century, cytologic analysis of the vomitus and lavage materials from the stomach was rather common. In 1858 Lionel S. Beale (14), in London, recommended examination for malignant cells in the vomitus when gastric carcinoma was suspected. This type of procedure was also very popular in Germany, as is attested by the works of Boas (25), Rosenbach (233), and Reineboth (227), and careful search for small fragments of neoplastic tissue, and occasionally isolated cells, was performed almost routinely, occasionally with success in diagnosing gastric carcinoma.

The first purely cytological work—that is, the inference of the existence of cancer from morphologic characteristics of individual cells—was done by Giovanni Marini (175) in 1909 at Bologna University in Italy. He conceived the idea that fresh material obtained by gastric lavage might contain better preserved malignant cells. By his pioneer use of tube lavage with an alkaline solution, he demonstrated malignant cells in thirty-two of thirty-seven gastric and esophageal carcinomas, a very surprising result in view of the use of unstained, unfixed material. The illustrations of Marini's work include a clear and unmistakable picture of a "tadpole" cell, *Geschwanzt* as he designated it, as well as other types of probably malignant cells.

This was the beginning of exfoliative cytology as we understand it today. However, the lack of an effective and practical staining method, such as that developed by Papanicolaou, and an undue emphasis on the significance of nonmalignant cells in various processes were largely responsible for the slow progress initially.

In 1911 Loeper and Binet (165), in Paris, reported the use of a saline lavage of the stomach that does not differ much from the method in use today. They extended Marini's observations by applying stains to the slides: hematoxylin-eosin and Toluidine Blue. But these investigators did not mention the number of cases studied or the accuracy of their cytologic diagnosis. A few years later, in 1914, Simon and Caussade (261) also reported very good results with cytology: twenty-four positive cytodiagnoses among twenty-five tumors.

The rapid progress of radiology and endoscopy for the next three decades led to a hiatus in the further development of gastrointestinal cytology. Only in the late 1940s, after the popularization of the Papanicolaou techniques, has exfoliative cytology of the gastrointestinal

TABLE 2.1
SOME HIGHLIGHTS IN THE EVOLUTION OF (GASTROINTESTINAL) CYTOLOGY AND OTHER DIAGNOSTIC METHODS

1590	Janssen invents the microscope (Holland)
1793	Mathew Baillie publishes the first edition of *The Morbid Anatomy of Some of the Most Important Parts of the Human Body* (London)
1839	T. Schwann enunciates his cell theory (Berlin)
1846	W. H. Walshe publishes *The Nature and Treatment of Cancer* (London)
1881	Billroth performs the first successful partial gastrectomy in a human (Germany)
1881	Mikulicz publishes a series of articles describing the first really successful gastroscope (Germany)
1895	Roentgen discovers the X ray (Germany)
1909	Marini publishes the first strictly "exfoliative cytology" work using gastric washings (Bologna, Italy)
1910	Barium sulphate becomes the standard contrast medium for gastric radiology (Germany)
1923	R. Schindler publishes his *Lehrbuch und Atlas der Gastroskopie* (Munich)
1928	Papanicolaou recognizes carcinoma cells exfoliated from the female genital tract (New York)
1939	R. A. Guttman (Paris) publishes his pioneer work on the radiological detection of small ulcerated gastric carcinomas
1941	Papanicolaou and Traut publish the classic paper "The Diagnostic Value of Vaginal Smears in Diagnosis of Uterine Cancer" (USA)
1946	Papanicolaou reports his initial experiences with gastric cytology (USA)
1948	Graham reintroduces saline washings (Marini's concept), using the Papanicolaou staining method (USA)
1949	Barr and Bertram describe sex chromatin, establishing the sexual dimorphism of mammalian nuclei (Canada)
1950	Uji introduces the first successful intragastric photographic instrument, the "gastrocamera" (Japan)
1958	The first gastroscope incorporating "fiber optics" is introduced by Hirschowitz and his colleagues (USA)
1962	The Japanese Gastroenterological Endoscopy Society defines "early gastric carcinoma" and establishes a useful macroscopical classification.
1964	The first successful direct-vision cytology through the new fibergastroscopes (Japan).

tract regained its place in the diagnostic armamentarium. During the 1950s, the contributions of Rubin et al. (238–46) and later of Raskin et al. (216–24) at the gastrointestinal cytology laboratory of the University of Chicago were most important in establishing reproducible and accurate washing techniques for gastrointestinal cytological diagnosis.

The work of Schade (250–52) in England, stressing the possibility of "early" diagnosis of superficial gastric carcinoma, also was highly significant. This study emphasized exfoliative cytology as the method of choice for mass surveys of selected asymptomatic population groups at risk, or as a mass survey tool in countries like Japan, Chile, and Germany, which have very high incidences of gastric carcinoma.

Important progress has recently been made possible by the introduction of new fiberscopes; with these remarkably safe and versatile instruments it has been possible to wash or brush minute and superficial lesions *under direct vision* (144–45, 147–48).

Readers interested in the historical developments that culminated in the late 1940s in Papanicolaou's first efforts in gastric cytology are referred to the excellent chapters on this subject in the monograph *Exfoliative Cytology of the Stomach* by Gibbs (88).

Part 2

Methodology in Gastrointestinal Exfoliative Cytology

3
Methods of Cell Collection

The large number of methods that have been proposed for cell collection in gastrointestinal diagnostic cytology attests to both the technical difficulties and the ingenuity applied in surmounting them. Unfortunately, no one method can claim absolute absence of sampling error, ease of performance, and complete acceptance by all patients—the ideal qualities of a good cell collection method.

Faced with this limitation, the cytopathologist must compromise and use the method with which he has most experience and diagnostic success. The same method, however, may not produce similar results in other hands. As will be emphasized frequently in this monograph, meticulous care and attention to details are essential to success in gastrointestinal cytology. As a result, cell collection must be done by well-trained and highly motivated cytotechnicians; the busy intern or nurse simply has not the time or the training for this task. In a questionnaire survey on the usefulness of gastric cytology, done in the United States in 1967 by Ackerman (1), it was noted that in the series reporting the most accurate results the cytological specimens were collected primarily under the supervision of gastroenterologists. Absence of a formal cytological team was deemed responsible for the low accuracy in six of eleven hospitals reporting low accuracy.

The recent availability of efficient and remarkably engineered fiberscopes that permit cytological sampling under direct vision has enormously facilitated cell collection from the esophagus and stomach, and has not reduced the detection rate (actually it has increased the success rate to nearly 100% when combined with biopsy). But the method will never be generally available because an experienced endoscopist is needed. In centers with such facilities, however, the method easily supersedes any other, and only those few patients in whom endoscopy is contraindicated will not benefit from it. Fortunately, the increasing availability of fiber endoscopes is greatly enlarging the use of endoscopy in gastroenterology, and before long these techniques should be available generally.

The wider use of duodenal drainage for cell collection from lesions in the pancreas, biliary tree, and duodenum should be encouraged. The technique of duodenal intubation is not difficult and it can be mastered in a few weeks by an interested technician. Fluoroscopic control, however, is a definite requirement. The availability of

safe and practical duodenoscopes probably will help with the application of the direct-vision principle in many cases.

The colon also remains a difficult area for cell collection; the cleansing of the bowel for this procedure is difficult and is not well tolerated by all patients, especially those with ulcerative colitis. The percentage of unsatisfactory results remains high (about 7% in the hands of our highly trained technicians). The new colonoscopes should facilitate collection of cells under direct vision.

Esophagus and Stomach

Washing Methods

Ordinarily, all that is required to prepare the patient is an overnight fast. If there is gross retention because of obstruction, the esophagus or stomach is cleansed before the fast by aspiration with an Ewald tube in the evening before the test, and the area is washed with isotonic saline or Ringer's solution until the returns are clear, to facilitate adequate exfoliation and help secure clear slides. It is helpful to remind the patient to withhold antacids and other medication.

With the patient sitting upright, a number 16 or 18 french rubber Levin tube is passed through the mouth into the esophagus by the cytotechnician. Mild lubrication of the tip of the tube with water is desirable. An attempt is always made to pass beyond any obstruction and then enter the stomach through the cardia.

Esophageal Washing. With the tip of the Levin tube located at the cardia, the patient is given approximately 100 ml of Ringer's solution to swallow slowly. As this fluid is swallowed, gentle aspiration with a 100-ml syringe is maintained. The material thus obtained represents a sampling of the entire esophagus.

After the esophageal swallow, the tube is withdrawn 3 to 5 cm. The area at this point is washed with 20 to 40 ml of Ringer's solution. This procedure is repeated at graduated levels until the upper esophagus is reached. A fluid return of approximately one-half of the amount swallowed is to be expected. If there is an obstruction, however, the aspirate will approximate the amount instilled. At the conclusion of the washing procedure, the tube is again passed into the stomach, and the gastric content is aspirated. The aspirated material is collected in 50-ml plastic centrifuge tubes immersed in an ice bath and is centrifuged immediately after the collection is completed (see section on Slide Preparation).

Gastric Washing. First the stomach is aspirated and the volume and the nature of the residual material are noted. With the patient in a sitting position, 300 ml of Ringer's solution are injected vigorously into the stomach with a 100-ml syringe, and aspiration and injection are quickly repeated over a 3- to 5-min period. The forceful movement of fluid tends to remove the mucous layer with entrapped cells, and it also increases the exfoliation of cells from the mucosa. The fluid then is aspirated in 50-ml increments and placed in plastic centrifuge tubes immersed in an ice bath, ready for immediate centrifugation. Three hundred milliliters of Ringer's solution are reinjected into the stomach and the patient is rotated to the left and right sides while vigorous introduction and withdrawal of the fluid are continued. Some technicians prefer 50-ml syringes for the injection and aspiration because this size requires less effort.

In our experience, about 7% of the gastric washings are unsatisfactory because of food retention (especially in pyloric obstruction) or too little exfoliation of cells; this is in close agreement with other authors, for example Rubin and Brandborg (241), who have reported 10% with the chymotrypsin method. In a comparative study, Foushee et al. (74) had about 22% unsatisfactory washings, without significant differences between saline washings and chymotrypsin lavage.

Direct-Vision Cytology

Since the Olympus GF-B Gastro-Fiberscope and EF Esophago-Fiberscope have been available, we perform direct-vision cytology at the time of endoscopy. Both the gastrofiberscope and the esophagofiberscope contain a channel within their shafts through which a flexible probe tipped with a nylon brush, a polyethylene tube, or a biopsy forceps may be passed (fig. 3.1a,b). The brush tip is 8 mm in length with a diameter of 3mm, and the closed cups of the forceps have a diameter of about 2 mm. The tips of both endoscopes can be flexed through an arc of 180° so that the brush or forceps can be accurately applied to the lesion. A major difference between the two instruments is the orientation of the objective lens. The esophagoscope gives a forward view, whereas the gastroscope makes visible a lateral field.

Direct-vision cytology is accomplished by either of two methods.

Washing. A polyethylene tube, provided by the manufacturer, is passed through the biopsy-cytology channel of the scope. Its tip can be maneuvered by proximal control and is easily seen in the field of view. A 100-ml syringe filled with Ringer's solution is attached to the tube, and a forceful jet is directed at the lesion, under direct vision and remote control. The lesion usually bleeds slightly, and this is an additional criterion that it has been accurately washed. After the instrument is withdrawn, the lavage fluid is recovered by intubating the patient with a Levin tube and aspirating the gastric contents. The aspirated material is processed as in the usual washing methods. It is important to note that if washing cytology is to be done, no antifoam agent should be used in preparing the patient for endoscopy.

Brushing. A nylon brush in the tip of a flexible spiral wire, provided by the manufacturer, is introduced through the cytology-biopsy channel of the scope. It can be maneuvered by proximal control so as to come into view. Then its tip can be advanced and pulled back gently several times, to brush the lesion. Since the brushing is done under direct vision, one can be sure the lesion has been accurately reached. The brush then is withdrawn and smeared on clear glass microscope slides. Usually three smears can be made from each of the two or three brushings (figs. 3.2 and 3.3).

We prefer the brushing method because: (*a*) it dispenses with the Levin intubation after endoscopy; (*b*) the smears are made immediately without the necessity of centrifugation, saving time; (*c*) the background in the microscopical field is much reduced, making the screening much easier and quicker for the technician; (*d*) an antifoam agent can be used before the endoscopic examination; (*e*) in the cases of stenosis of the pylorus or cardia, lavage under direct vision is frequently unsatisfactory, whereas brushing remains feasible and yields good material; (*f*) washing under direct vision requires three intubations—a preliminary but thorough washing to clean the stomach, the endoscopy intubation, and the intubation to aspirate the cell-rich fluid (132). This increases the time spent, and reduces the patient's tolerance for the procedure.

We disagree with the view (241) that "cells abraded directly from a lesion, unlike those spontaneously exfoliated, often are morphologically confusing and may lead to inaccurate diagnoses." First, the cells they obtain usually are exfoliated by the chymotrypsin lavage and are not shed "spontaneously." Second, we find the cells collected by the brush so well preserved that their morphology is easier to study. Fibroblasts, in our experience, are easily recognized (209).

Other Cell Collection Methods: Stomach

Mechanical Methods. Since Hemmeter (107) in 1889 described an abrasive instrument for diagnosing gastric carcinoma, many devices have been utilized. We will briefly describe those employed in the past or now in use in selected laboratories.

1. The *Zelltüpfsonde* of Henning and Witte (109, 110) consists of a semirigid tube provided with a steel wire carrying at the distal end a detachable foam-rubber sponge, which can enter the stomach within the cover of the tube. More recently, this instrument has been modified to permit abrasion of the antrum under fluoroscopic control. It has not been impressive in its sampling accuracy in gastric carcinoma. The frequent need for fluoroscopic control also makes it less simple to use. In a series of 139 tumors of the body and antrum of the stomach (112), definite or probable positive results were obtained in 72% of the tumors of the body of the stomach and in 64% of the antral tumors. In the opinion of Schade (250), the instrument is more useful for the study of diffuse inflammatory lesions of the stomach.

2. The *gastric abrasive balloon* of Cooper and Papanicolaou (58, 71, 72, 199, 274) consists of a double-lumen rubber tube with a thin rubber balloon fastened to the distal end. The balloon is encased in a wide-meshed silk netting. One lumen of the tube is used for inflating the balloon and the other for aspirating gastric contents and for lavage. The balloon is inflated within the stomach and with its surrounding net is moved across the mucosal surface by direct manipulation of the proximal end of the tube and by natural peristaltic action, causing abrasive exfoliation of cells. After withdrawal, the balloon is rinsed in Ringer's solution and the suspension is centrifuged. Smears are made as usual from the sediment. Sampling of the antrum is not reliable with this instrument, and so Panico (198) and Rubin (238,

246) devised antrum balloons to overcome this difficulty. As with most instruments of this category, the sampling error in gastric carcinoma is high and does not compare with the washing methods. Bruinsma has adapted such balloons for use in the esophagus (37). The need for local anesthesia of the pharynx and palate in some patients is another inconvenience and adds a remote risk to the procedure.

3. Ayre's *gastric brush* (10) and the all-plastic retractable brush of Nieburgs et al. (189) are easily rotated inside the stomach, and sampling of the body probably is adequate; but the instruments do not reach the antrum, which again prevents reliable sampling of cells from this area. The presence of esophageal varices contraindicates the use of the brush, and accidental gastric biopsies have been reported (235).

4. Cabre-Fiol's *mandrel tube* (42–44), used in Barcelona, is an ingenious combination of a washing and an abrasion technique. It consists of a radiopaque, double-lumen plastic tube provided with a steel wire ending in a rubber tip to avoid traumatic punctures. Attached to the wire is a tuft of nylon thread loops which is placed into a soft cylinder, 4 cm long and 1 cm in diameter. Exfoliation is done under fluoroscopy by moving the steel wire with the nylon thread tuft back and forth against the gastric walls. The stomach then is washed with ice-cold saline solution through an additional tube opening. An accuracy rate comparable to that of the regular washing methods has been reported by investigators using this method. A positive cytodiagnosis was made in 280 of 316 patients with gastric cancer, a detection rate of 88.6% (288). Again, the need for fluoroscopy makes the method less simple.

Lavage with "Mucolytic" Agents. Many physicians advocate adding chemical agents to the washing solution in an attempt to digest the gastric mucus and facilitate exfoliation, thereby decreasing sampling error. The first method devised was the buffered papain solution of Rosenthal and Traut (234). It was tested in our laboratory by Rubin and Benditt (240), but the variability in cell preservation led them to use alpha-chymotrypsin. Chymotrypsin is added to the lavage fluid (7 mg of crystalline alpha-chymotrypsin per 300 to 500 ml of 0.1 M acetate buffer at pH 5.6), or the patient may drink it in a glass of water 30 min before lavage with the acetate buffer solution, "short chymotrypsin method" (34). Lavage with Ringer's solution immediately followed by the antral abrasive balloon was at that time the standard cell collection method in Rubin's laboratory. Hence it is understandable that he considered the chymotrypsin method easier and less complicated. Actually, no comparison was made between lavage with Ringer's solution only and the chymotrypsin method. Cellularity usually seemed to be increased, but the overall accuracy in gastric carcinoma was not significantly greater. Later, Raskin preferred the simple Ringer's or saline washing method first developed by Graham, Ulfelder, and Green (99) in 1948.

In the experience of Jensen and Schade (124), the use of chymotrypsin in a series of fifty patients with pernicious anemia was not advantageous. More recently, Yamada (302) in Japan reported in vitro studies showing a significant increase in cell exfoliation with higher concentrations of chymotrypsin, as well as clinical studies (303) claiming increased accuracy levels in gastric carcinoma. Brandborg, Tankersley, and Uyeda (35) studied two hundred patients by both "low" and "high" concentrations of chymotrypsin, the sequence of the tests being randomly assigned, and claimed a better yield of diagnostic cells with the "high" (about 5 mg per 100 ml) dose. However, overall cancer detection was not enhanced by increasing the concentration of chymotrypsin.

Brandborg and Wenger (36), Rubin and Brandborg (241), Klayman et al. (140, 141), MacDonald et al. (171), and Seppala (256) have reported good results with the method. Many discrepancies in results probably are due to different methods of reporting. The most important problem is the failure to accurately report the number of cases in which the initial test was unsatisfactory and no repeat test was possible. In the experience of Rubin and Brandborg (241) and Brandborg and Wenger (36), approximately 10% of patients may require repeat examination because of inadequate sampling. In our own experience, about 7% of gastric washings are unsatisfactory. So far no case of gastric brushing has been unsatisfactory in more than two hundred examinations performed.

In an interesting paper (35), Brandborg, Tankersley, and Uyeda made a blind comparison between saline and chymotrypsin washing methods; the latter was considered superior because of the increased cellularity of the smears. But the "positive rate" in the presence of carcinoma—the crucial test—was the same in both methods.

Saburi et al. (247) reported an ingenious modification of the chymotrypsin lavage method—adding to the lavage fluid a radiopaque water-soluble iodine derivative (3-acetylamino-2,4,6-triiodobenzoic acid). Selective washings of suspicious lesions were obtained under fluoroscopic control through a specially devised rubber tube less flexible than the ordinary Levin tube (allowing better control of its position). The concentration of chymotrypsin also was high: 5 mg per dl of solution. By this method, 146 positive diagnoses, or 96.7%, were obtained in 151 proved cancers. A hematoxylin-eosin staining method was used.

In conclusion, we have little doubt that the washing methods are the easiest and simplest techniques for "blind" collection of cells, an opinion shared by Jensen and Schade (124), Brandborg, Taniguchi, and Rubin (34), and Raskin, Kirsner, and Palmer (216). It is also our opinion that the washing technique probably is the method of choice in mass surveys for gastric carcinoma in countries with a very high incidence of such tumors. This will be discussed further in chapter 9. In the *clinical evaluation* of patients suspected of having gastric carcinoma, it is superseded by the direct-vision method, with its smaller sampling error, when an endoscopy team is available and integrated with the cytology team, as will be discussed in chapter 8.

Duodenum, Biliary Passages, and Pancreas

The method developed by Raskin et al. (224) is utilized with minor modifications.

Intubation. The patient fasts overnight. The Dreiling tube is passed orally to 45 cm, with the metal olive situated at the level of the cardia. The patient lies with head elevated in the left lateral decubitus position and *slowly* swallows 15 cm of additional tubing. The excess tubing lies along the greater curvature. The patient then sits up and bends forward at the waist, taking several deep inspirations. This helps the tip of the tube enter the antrum as the anterior wall of the stomach falls away from the posterior wall. The patient then lies in the right lateral decubitus position for 5 min and then on the back for 3 or 4 min, during which time 10–15 cm of additional tubing is advanced, after which the position is checked fluoroscopically. The tip of the tube is placed at the midportion of the descending part of the duodenum, entirely to the right side of the spine. Drainage is initiated with the patient lying on his back on a horizontal examining table. Utilizing the method described above, duodenal intubation is usually completed in about 15 min.

In Raskin's words (224), the two salient features of this method of intubation are the left lateral decubitus position and the next step, bending forward. Placing the patient on the left side prevents the tube from impinging on the lesser curvature, particularly in cascade configurations of the stomach. As the patient bends forward and takes several deep breaths, the tube, which is under some tension and recoils because of the excess length, will slide into the antrum. Peristalsis will then rapidly carry the tip through the pyloric canal. Lippman (163), in 1914, appreciated the importance of having the patient lean forward as a means of introducing the tube into the antrum. Although he did not utilize the left lateral decubitus, his method was rapid and accurate; unfortunately, it was only one of many advocated and never received adequate recognition.

The standard procedures as described by Lyon (167, 168) and Cantor (47) usually require 1 to 2 hr for intubation. The studies of Lake (156) in 1940 did much to disprove the theory that the weight or shape of the tip of the tube was a major factor in successful intubation. Approximately fifty gastroduodenal tubes had been devised in an endeavor to enhance passage. Lake attempted 396 intubations utilizing rubber tubes without tips (Levin tube) and with weighted tips up to 10 gm (Einhorn tube). Weighted tubes all reached the duodenum in approximately the same time, but the lighter Levin tube was not quite as fast. Regardless of the type of tube used, 66% of the 396 subjects were successfully intubated in 30 min; 20% required up to 2 hr, and 14% of the attempts were unsuccessful.

Collection of Duodenal Aspirate. The purpose of the double-lumen tube is to drain the alkaline duodenal content separately from the acid gastric secretion. Not only does gastric sediment, which contains respiratory and esophageal epithelial cells, interfere with the cellular study of the duodenal fluid, but neutralization of the alkaline pancreatic secretion would invalidate the secretin test portion of the examination. Pancreatic se-

cretion should not be collected until adequate gastric drainage has been completed. Introducing 200 cc of air through the gastric lumen, followed by aspiration, with the patient inclined toward the right lateral position, will facilitate complete emptying of the stomach. The gastric and duodenal tubes are then connected to a constant vacuum pump (Gomco) with pressure of 120 mm Hg. The gastric juice is carried directly into a collecting jar and is discarded, but the duodenal aspirate is diverted by a simple trap which consists of 50-cc plastic centrifuge tubes immersed in an ice bath. Occasional pH determinations of both drainages are made with litmus paper during the control collection to ensure continuous independent drainage. Occasionally, inadvertently placing the most distal gastric openings in the duodenum may yield an alkaline juice on the gastric lumen. Similarly, the continuous presence of acid in the duodenal aspirate indicates incomplete emptying of the stomach or failure to place the most distal gastric openings in the antrum. These problems are quickly remedied by minor adjustments of the tube.

Once proper drainage has been assured, a 10-min control sample is collected and saved. Secretin, in a dose of 1 unit per kg of body weight, is then injected intravenously. Before injection a routine intradermal sensitivity test is performed. The pancreatic secretion is collected for ½ hr in three 10-min samples. The purpose of dividing the postsecretin collection into three equal parts is to determine the maximum pancreatic response. At the conclusion of the drainage, the duodenal aspirate is centrifuged for 10 min at 5,000 rpm. The supernatant fluid of the three 10-min specimens is decanted and saved for chemical analysis. The sediment is immediately smeared on "frosted" glass slides and fixed in 95% ethyl alcohol, and subsequently is stained by the modified Papanicolaou method (see section on Slide Preparation). At the termination of the drainage a simple saline lavage of the duodenum and distal stomach is performed for cytologic purposes.

Secretin. The availability of secretin free of factors which cause adverse reactions and of relatively constant potency has facilitated the study immeasurably. Heretofore, commercial secretin produced an occasional reaction and even death, and was of questionable stability. No systemic reactions have been observed in this series. Occasionally patients develop a slight erythematous zone around the site of intradermal injection. Raskin et al. (224) observed one patient with malignant reticuloendotheliosis of the skin who developed a giant urticarial wheal at the site of the intradermal test, necessitating termination of the examination.

Pancreozymin-Cholecystokinin (Cecekin). In selected cases, especially when there may be biliary tract stones, an injection of Cecekin is given before the secretin test. A qualitative determination of "B" bile is made if dark bile is obtained within several minutes after the injection. The material obtained is centrifuged and the sediment is prepared as described above for cytological examination. In addition, a slide is usually prepared, without fixation, to demonstrate calcium bilirubinate or cholesterol crystals, with the phase microscope or with the standard illumination with the diaphragm halfway closed (see chap. 11).

Colon

The method of Raskin (222, 223) is used with minimal modifications.

Preparation of the Patient. The preparation of the patient is as important as the diagnostic lavage. It is most advantageous to place the patient on a low residue diet as soon as the procedure is planned. Liquids are allowed for breakfast on the day of the examination. Colonic cytology should not be scheduled within 24 hr of a barium enema but should be deferred for at least two days. During this period the colon should be cleansed with isotonic saline solution or with tap-water enemas. At approximately noon of the day before the planned cytologic procedure, a strong cathartic is administered. Two ounces of castor oil is very effective, but in some individuals castor oil produces cramping severe enough to cause fainting. In recent years, particularly in the elderly, we have been utilizing a contact laxative called Dulcolax.[1] The preferred dose of Dulcolax is four tablets at noon and four tablets at 4 P.M.

At 8 A.M. on the day of the examination cleansing enemas should be initiated. The foot of the bed is elevated on 12-in "shock blocks." The patient is positioned on his left side, head down, with his thighs flexed. Each

cleansing enema should consist of 2,500 cc of isotonic saline solution. Most nurses trained in traditional procedures are reluctant to give large quantities of fluid because they assume that severe cramping will occur. In the absence of a stricture of the left colon, or ulcerative colitis, the patient usually can retain a large quantity of fluids, as the major portion will gravitate to the splenic flexure. Ordinary enemas of approximately 500 ml frequently will cause cramping and distension of the rectal ampulla when the patient lies supine. Once the cleansing enema has been slowly instilled, the patient rotates to his back for approximately 5 min while remaining in the Trendelenburg position, and then turns to the right side. The irrigating solution now probably has traveled to the hepatic flexure and ascending colon. In a thin person the fluid is palpated easily in the right colon. After reclining for 10 min in the right lateral position, the patient goes to the bathroom and evacuates the bowel. The nurse or attendant examines the contents before flushing the toilet. The quantity of solid fecal material is noted. A second and third enema of similar proportions are then given. Frequently the third enema will return clear except for a yellowish tint and mucus shreds. These two findings are acceptable indications of adequate preparation for a diagnostic enema. If amorphous sediment is present in the bottom of the toilet bowl or bedpan, another enema is required. A member of the cytology team inspects the final cleansing enema before the patient is considered adequately prepared.

Special efforts are required to cleanse the large bowel in patients with ulcerative colitis or stricture of the left colon and in those with previous resections of the left colon or of the ileocecal valve. In ulcerative colitis, the lumen of the left colon frequently is narrowed, and the walls are thickened and cannot readily be distended. Another limitation in ulcerative colitis is caused by adherence of large amounts of mucus and feces to the diseased bowel mucosa. In spite of cooperation the patient frequently experiences so much discomfort in retaining 2,500 ml of fluid that smaller quantities and more numerous enemas are required. There is also the potential hazard of producing a clinical exacerbation with cathartics in ulcerative colitis; hence Dulcolax often is preferred in these patients also. It is sometimes difficult, depending upon the degree of narrowing, to adequately cleanse the left colon above the level of a stricture produced by diverticulitis or carcinoma. There usually is

---

1. Dulcolax (brand of bisacodyl), is a contact laxative effective orally and by suppository, supplied by Geigy Pharmaceuticals. Similar preparations undoubtedly will serve as well.

stasis of feces and frequently mild dilatation of the bowel above the point of narrowing. A cleansing enema consequently fails to penetrate far beyond the narrowed segment and seemingly always leaves liquid feces behind. Therefore multiple enemas, perhaps as many as ten, may be necessary to adequately prepare the colon for cytologic study. In such instances, though not commonly, two days may be necessary for bowel preparation.

In patients with congestive heart failure who are receiving diuretics and digitalis, tap water is preferred to isotonic saline for cleansing enemas. Because of salt absorption, patients with congestive heart failure may experience a mild increase in respiratory symptoms following the procedure. Similarly, although we have had no experience, it seems desirable to use saline solution in patients with megacolon, since the literature records instances of hyponatremia and circulatory collapse when such patients are given copious tap-water enemas.

The Diagnostic Enemas

The procedure should be performed on a conventional proctoscopic table. The table should be tilted as far forward (down) as possible, and if possible the sigmoidoscope is passed to a level at least 25 cm above the anal verge. This is beyond the rectosigmoid junction; the sharp angulation of the colon at 15 cm sometimes acts as a physiologic obstruction to the free flow of fluid. A standard no. 28 Ewald tube then is threaded through the sigmoidoscope and the tip of the rubber tube is extended another 10 cm or so beyond the proctoscope by gentle pushing and occasional twirling. If difficulty is encountered in passing the Ewald tube, particularly if the 25-cm level has not been reached with the sigmoidoscope, two maneuvers may help. One requires the use of an air insufflator similar to the type utilized for air contrast barium enemas. The upper rectum and lower sigmoid can be gently distended with several bagfuls of air. Sometimes this is enough to separate the walls and allow the Ewald tube to proceed. If this procedure fails, 200 or 300 ml of the diagnostic wash fluid may be allowed to flow slowly through the Ewald tube and open the lumen. It is important to get beyond the rectosigmoid junction, not only to allow the diagnostic enema to enter rapidly, but, more important, to facilitate collection of the fluid on return from the right side of the bowel.

Once the Ewald tube has been projected approximately 10 cm beyond the sigmoidoscope, the metal instru-

ment is withdrawn, leaving the rubber tube in the colon. The tube then is connected to a canister holding 800 ml of normal physiologic saline solution at 36° C. Saline solution should always be used for the *diagnostic* enema in spite of a history of cardiac disease, since it is best for cell preservation. There will be a rapid flow of fluid with no sensation to the patient, since he is in a head-down position. When the cannister is empty, the tube is clamped and the proctoscopic table is righted. The lower portion of the table (the thigh and knee rest portion) is extended, making a flat surface. The patient then lies on his right side so that the fluid may gravitate more easily from the splenic flexure to the hepatic flexure. After a few minutes the patient is positioned on his back so that the fluid may fill the ascending colon and finally the cecum.

All four quadrants of the abdomen then are vigorously massaged by the operator for 3 min, with emphasis upon the quadrant containing the suspected colon lesion. The Ewald tube then is unclamped and the diagnostic enema fluid is siphoned off through an ordinary coarse-mesh tea strainer into a 1-l beaker, two-thirds submerged in an ice bath. The enema fluid will return in gushes corresponding to the peristaltic contractions of the colon. As long as 10 min may be required to recover 500 ml of the 800-ml diagnostic wash. Drainage may be enhanced if the patient lies on his left side. Occasionally, the gentle introduction of air into the descending colon will free some of the entrapped fluid.

Always use a strainer of large mesh. Too fine a strainer will trap diagnostic cells in small pieces of mucus.

At the conclusion of the first enema, a second diagnostic enema is given by restoring the proctoscopic table to its original position, lowering the head and introducing an additional 800 ml of fluid. The identical maneuvers and positions are repeated. Usually this enema will bring down some of the retained fluid from the first enema, and returns exceeding 800 ml in the second lavage are not unusual. The second enema usually contains less sediment and more diagnostic cells.

Slide Preparation

The aspirates of esophageal, gastric, and colonic washes are centrifuged for 5 min at 5,000 rpm, and the duodenal drainage aspirate is centrifuged for 10 min at 5,000 rpm, in 50-ml plastic centrifuge tubes. After the supernatant fluid is discarded (as was stated previously, the supernatant fluid of the duodenal drainage is saved for the bicarbonate determination), the button of sediment is lifted from the bottom of the centrifuge tube with fine metal spatulas and smeared on "frosted" glass slides. (The "frosted" surface facilitates adherence of the material to the surface without the use of albumin; there is no "fallout" when the slides are placed in the fixative.) It is preferable to use as many as six pairs of slides so that the material is deposited as a thin layer. Reading time is shortened and diagnostic accuracy improved with thin smears. Small flecks of blood frequently will be concentrated in the center of the centrifuged sediment tube. These areas should always be smeared, because they often contain large groups of malignant cells, occasionally serving as "microbiopsies."

We have had no experience with the use of membrane filters for cell concentration; this may be a satisfactory technique, especially if "mucolytic" agents are used in the washes.

Immediate fixation by immersion in a solution of 95° ethylalcohol is the final step. Fifteen minutes is an adequate fixation time.

TABLE 3.1

SPECIMEN PROCESSING FLOW CHART

Patient Preparation [a]	Cell Collection	Cytopathology	Clerical
Day before:			
Clear liquid supper	Washing or direct-vision brushing	Staining	Filing
With gastric wash; suspend antacids or other medication	Ice-bath collection of aspirates	Screening	
	Centrifugation	Diagnosis	
Day of examination:			
8-hr fast	Slide preparation		
Withhold all medication by mouth	Immediate fixation		

[a] Colonic washing requires special preparation (see text), and direct-vision brushing is part of the complete endoscopic examination.

4

Staining Methods

Papanicolaou's Staining Method

Meticulous care and personal familiarity with a special staining method are more important in obtaining the best results than any particular qualities claimed for the staining methods (88). For gastrointestinal cytology, hematoxylin and eosin have been used by Saburi et al. (247), Pappenheim's stain by Henning and Witte (110), and May-Grunwald-Giemsa by Lopes Cardozo (166) and Kasugai (132, 133). Nevertheless, the properties developed by Papanicolaou (200–202) in his method of staining have been extremely satisfactory for gastrointestinal cytology. Even in very thick smears the individual cell takes up the staining very well and is easily recognized even in thick clumps or large amounts of mucus. In the United States, this is the standard staining method in exfoliative cytology.

There are many minor modifications of Papanicolaou's original methods, and the following technique has been very satisfactory in our laboratory.

After the fixative bath, the slides are passed through the following sequence:

1. Alcoholic solution of celloidin for 2 min (skip if using "frosted" slides)
2. 70% ethanol for 2 min
3. Distilled water for 2 min
4. Distilled water for 1 min
5. Harris's hematoxylin for 2 min
6. Tap water with $LiCO_3$ for 1 min
7. Tap water with $LiCO_3$ for ½ min
8. Differentiate in 1% HCl for 10 sec (5 dips)
9. Tap water with $LiCO_3$ for 1 min
10. Tap water with $LiCo_3$ for 2 min
11. Tap water with $LiCO_3$ for 5 min
12. 70% ethanol for 1 min
13. 95% ethanol for 1 min
14. Stain in Orange G (OG-6) for 2 min
15. 95% ethanol for 1 min
16. 95% ethanol for 1 min
17. Stain in Papanicolaou's stain EA-36 for 3 min
18. 95% ethanol for 1 min
19. 95% ethanol for 1 min
20. 100% ethanol (changed daily) for 5 min
21. Clear in Xylol for 5 min
22. Mount in Permount

A few comments about our technique: in step 1, using a 2% ethyl alcohol solution of celloidin instead of coating the slides with Mayer's albumin has been found advantageous, because it allows easier smearing on the thoroughly dry clear glass. This step can be omitted if the smears are made on "frosted" slides because cells adhere to this type of slide extremely well. For smearing the material from the brush used on direct-vision collection we prefer the clear glass slides (frosted only on one end, used for writing the date of collection, name of patient, or any other pertinent information). With the use of celloidin and frosted slides we have decreased almost to zero the incidence of "floaters," and we have not had any false-positive cases by contamination of one slide by another.

We prefer to use EA-36 prepared in our laboratory, which is equivalent to the EA-50 commercial preparation available.

We use the same formula of Durfee (in Koss, 151), as follows:

Formula for EA-36
1. Eosin Y   10gm
2. Bismarck Brown Y   10 gm
3. Light green SF, yellowish   10 gm
4. Distilled water   300 ml
5. 95% alcohol (ethyl)   2,000 ml
6. Phosphotungstic acid   4 gm
7. Saturated lithium carbonate solution (in distilled water) 20 drops

Procedure:
1. Stock Solution no. 1
   Prepare separate 10% solutions in each of the stains as follows:
   a) 10 gm Eosin Y in 100 ml distilled water
   b) 10 gm Bismarck Brown Y in 100 ml distilled water
   c) 10 gm Light green SF in 100 ml distilled water.
2. Mix (for 2,000 ml stain):
   a) 50 ml Eosin Y stock no. 1
   b) 10 ml Bismarck Brown Y stock no. 1
   c) 12.5 ml Light green SF stock no. 1.
3. Add 95% alcohol to make up 2,000 ml.
4. Add:
   a) 4 gm phosphotungstic acid
   b) 20 drops saturated lithium carbonate solution.

5. Mix well. Store solution in dark brown, tightly capped bottles.
   For use: Use full strength; filter before using.

Shorr Polychromic S3

We use the following recipe, taken from Durfee in Koss's book (151), after minor modifications:

Ethyl alcohol (50%)	100 ml
Biebrich Scarlet (water solution)	0.5 gm
Orange G	0.25 gm
Fast-green FCF	0.075 gm
Phosphotungstic acid c.p.	0.5 gm
Phosphomolybdic acid c.p.	0.5 gm
Glacial acetic acid	1.0 ml

The solution should not be used until all the ingredients have dissolved completely.

1. Fix, while wet, in 95% ethyl alcohol. Fixation for 1 or 2 min is adequate. More recently, we added dimethylsulfoxide (DMSO) to a final concentration of 1%.
2. Stain for approximately 3 min in solution S3.
3. Carry through 70% and 95% ethanol, dipping slide ten times in each solution.
4. Dip ½ min in absolute ethanol.
5. Clear in xylol and mount.

Acridine-Orange Fluorescence Method

We again use the recipe of Koss and Durfee (151):

Method of Bertalanffy (pH6): Preparation of Solutions

Acridine-Orange Stock Solution. Prepare 0.1% aqueous stock solution of a good quality Acridine Orange. Store indefinitely in refrigerator.

Phosphate Buffer—pH 6. The phosphate buffer is a combination of M/15 potassium dihydrophosphate and M/15 sodium phosphate mixed in proportion to pH 6.

The solutions are prepared by dissolving 9.072 gm potassium dihydrophosphate (KH_2PO_4) in 1,000 ml distilled water, and 9.465 gm sodium phosphate (Na_2HPO_4) in 1,000 ml distilled water. To obtain the buffer, mix 230 ml potassium dihydrophosphate solution with 40 ml sodium phosphate solution.

Calcium chloride is used for differentiation in M/10 solution. It is prepared by dissolving 11.099 gm calcium choride in 1,000 ml distilled water. All these solutions will keep indefinitely even at room temperature.
Procedure:

1. Hydrate rapidly through graded ethyl alcohol solutions—80%, 70%, 50% to distilled water.
2. Rinse briefly in 1% acetic acid solution.
3. Wash in distilled water.
4. Stain 3 min in 0.01% stock Acridine Orange in phosphate buffer solution (one part A.O. stock to nine parts of phosphate buffer).
5. Transfer at least 1 min to phosphate buffer to remove excess dye. If batches of slides are processed, they may remain in buffer for several hours while they are examined successively.
6. Differentiate 1 to 2 min in M/10 calcium chloride until nuclei (especially of leukocytes) show bright green fluorescence. The time for differentiation can be standardized by trial.
7. Rinse with phosphate buffer by using a polyethylene wash bottle.
8. Mount wet, using a few drops of buffer under coverslip, and examine.

The time of the procedure is approximately 6 to 7 min. After microscopic examination, slides can be destained by placing them in 50% ethyl alcohol and then restained by the Papanicolaou technique or some other method.

5
Reporting the Results

After the cytotechnicians have completed the screening, the specimens are reviewed by the physician-cytopathologist in charge of the laboratory. Usually, special attention is paid only to the areas selected by the screeners, and for this purpose we prefer to use small circles drawn with water-removable ink. With this technique, slides can easily be converted into "unknown" slides to be re-screened by students. A photographic record of the best cytological fields is obtained as soon as possible to avoid stain fading or losses by breakage or misplacement.

After the slides are reviewed by the cytopathologist, a diagnosis is made and recorded in the laboratory's log book. The report is transcribed on special laboratory result sheets that are incorporated in the patients' charts. Whenever possible, the report states simply that malignant cells were either present ("positive" report) or absent ("negative" report) in the specimen. In our ex-

ber of cases in which retrospective study of the specimens in the group with negative report and positive followup revealed cells that were "suspicious" but not diagnostic of malignancy ("reader's error"). The final diagnosis in patients with a "class III" or "suspicious for malignancy" report in some reported series is noted in table 5.1. The percentage of proved cancers varies widely, according to the cytologist's confidence in the morphologic criteria of malignancy.

Another disadvantage of the class III or suspicious category report is that it obviates accurate calculation of the specificity of the positive report. If such reports were included in the positive category, the specificity of such positive reports would decrease considerably. If all are excluded, the true clinical picture may not be represented because many "suspicious" reports will be treated by the clinician as "positive."

TABLE 5.1

ANALYSIS OF FOLLOWUP OF CLASS III OR SUSPICIOUS REPORTS IN GASTROINTESTINAL CYTOLOGY

Author	Organ Studied and Method	No. of Class III or Suspicious Reports	Followup Showed Malignancy	Followup Showed No Malignancy
Johnson et al. (126)	Esophageal Washing	37	30 (81%)	7
Seybolt, Papanicolaou, and Cooper (257)	Gastric abrasive balloon	48	22 (45%)	26
Messelt (181)	Esophagoscopy swabs	23	18 (78%)	5
Umiker et al. (282)	Gastric chymotrypsin lavage	13	9 (69%)	4
Thabet and Knoerschild (275)	Colon washings and Millipore filtration	9	8 (88%)	1
Miller et al. (183)	Colonic washings	6	1 (16%)	5
Foushee et al. (74)	Esophageal and gastric washings	31	10 (33%)	21

perience, the use of a "suspicious" category, class III of Papanicolaou (200), is not advisable. It does not add anything to the clinical evaluation of symptomatic and selected patients, because the suspicion of gastrointestinal cancer already has been the main indication for the cytological examination. We find that it is possible, in the vast majority of instances, to decide whether the cells originate in a benign or a malignant lesion. This attitude is supported by our very small percentage of false-positive reports and also by the very small num-

As is emphasized elsewhere in this book, the main source of false-negative reports is *sampling error*. This sampling error is the basis of our frequent request for a repeat examination whenever the sampling is less than optimal. We do not think that this source of error can be excluded in any negative report; it should never outweigh clinical suspicion or exclude further investigation (210).

Occasionally, very atypical cells are present but on detailed review of the specimens not enough criteria are met to justify a positive report. It is our policy to report such an examination as negative, to note the presence of such atypical yet benign cells, and to suggest a repeat cytological examination. This situation happens most frequently in the presence of healing benign gastric ulcer, duodenal ulcer, and chronic ulcerative colitis. We agree with Fullmer et al. (78) that a realistic nomenclature of such atypias (dyskaryosis) is needed, but clinicians should be oriented to the significance of such cellular changes and not associate them with the old reports of "suspicious" of cancer. Long-term prospective studies of such cellular alterations will be of great importance.

The presence of other benign but probably significant cellular changes, such as the "bland" cells of atrophic gastritis or fibroblasts and Langhans's cells associated with granulomatous inflammatory changes also is included in the report. However, caution is frequently advised in interpreting such cellular changes because of their low specificity.

In the positive report, an attempt is made to delineate four main types of malignant tumors on the basis of the cellular morphology (see chaps. 14 and 15 for analysis of the criteria used): squamous cell carcinoma, adenocarcinoma, undifferentiated carcinoma, and malignant lymphoma. Further subdivision of any of these principal categories of neoplasia seems unwarranted.

In the absence of evidence of adequate exfoliation (amount of diagnostic cells) and of excellent morphological evidence of good preservation of the cells, the examination is reported as unsatisfactory and a repeat study is strongly suggested. This precaution is of paramount importance to avoid any undue sense of security given by a negative report issued in the presence of less than optimal cellular material. This policy is particularly important in gastric washing cytology, where a significant number of malignant tumors are in the distal antrum and are associated with retention of food and gastric content, which often leads to poor cytological material. Unfortunately, in a significant number of instances the examination is not repeated, thus decreasing the overall accuracy of the cytologic method. This is often true in colonic cytology because of the difficulty of completely cleansing the colon.

Not infrequently authors omit data on the exact number of unsatisfactory tests, achieving a spuriously high "accuracy" rate. Others provide such data but do not include them in the tabulation of the results, causing similar spuriously high percentages of correct diagnoses.

In cancer detection, it is more important to repeat an unsatisfactory test than a negative test.

Followup of Positive and Negative Reports

It is extremely important to secure adequate followup data on every patient examined. The followup of the positive report will reveal the usually small percentage of cases in which no cancer was detected (false-positive cases). The identification of false-negative cases is possible only by adequate followup months or years after the cytological study. A series with a large number of negative reports without followup data has little value, and the detection rate (usually referred to as "accuracy rate") of cancer may be much lower than stated. Some large series of gastric cytology lack a clear statement about the duration and the completeness of the followup.

In this book we have included only those patients with histologically proved cancer or with negative followup extending for *at least* one year and often longer; that is, the patient continued to attend our hospital and outpatient departments and no cancer of the gastrointestinal tract was discovered during this period.

Specificity and Sensitivity of Results

The specificity and the sensitivity of the results are the two important aspects in analyzing any diagnostic procedure in clinical medicine. Specificity is defined as the percentage of abnormal values caused by the respective pathological processes. The more specific a determined abnormal value, the more it helps in the management of the particular patient. Sensitivity is defined as the percentage of patients with a pathological process associated with respectively abnormal values. The sensitivity of a clinical test determines its general clinical usefulness and is independent of the specificity of any individual value. A test with low diagnostic sensitivity for a neoplastic process obviously will have limited or no value in cancer diagnosis.

In the diagnostic cytologic procedures described here, such an analysis is readily feasible because, for all practical purposes, only two values are utilized: the positive report for malignant cells and the negative report. The quotient of the number of patients with positive reports divided by the number of patients with proved cancer provides the cancer-diagnosis sensitivity of the method. For example, of 334 patients with adenocarcinoma of the stomach, 259 had a positive cytodiagnosis; this indicates a sensitivity quotient of 0.775; more easily expressed as 77.5%. This figure usually is referred to in the literature as the "accuracy" rate, and indicates that 77.5% of all gastric carcinomas are detected by the washing cytology of the stomach as performed in our laboratory. This is a reasonably high detection rate and the test should therefore be clinically useful. But, to be clinically useful in a particular case, an individual abnormal value must have specificity. The specificity of the positive cytodiagnosis is determined by the quotient of the total number of positive reports divided by the number of patients confirmed to have cancer of the organ studied (usually by histological proof, only exceptionally by clinical course). Returning to the example of washing cytology of the stomach: of 293 positive reports, 288 were proved correct, a specificity quotient of 0.982; in other words, 98.2% of the positive reports were correct (see tables 7.1 and 1.2). Any patient with a positive cytodiagnosis has an almost 100% chance of having carcinoma, and the result of the test can be used with confidence approaching that of a positive histological diagnosis.

meaningless because it is influenced by the proportion of cases with cancer in relation to the total number of patients studied. For example, if 15 of 20 positive reports are proved to be correct, the true specificity of the positive report is *only* 75% and the clinician should be aware of such low specificity. If the cytologist indicates that false-positive results are *only one per thousand* in his laboratory because his five false-positive reports were found in 5,000 patients without cancer, a false impression of the specificity of the positive report is provided. In table 5.2 we have tabulated the true specificity values of the positive report of several papers found in the literature which did not use class III or "suspicious" reports.

A corollary of such erroneous analysis of the data is the improper emphasis on the negative report. The same cytologist claiming a one per thousand false-positive rate will claim a 99.99 "accuracy" of his negative report; of 5,000 negative reports, only five, or one per thousand, were falsely negative. However, even if the detection rate of his method were only 80%, the patient with cancer and a negative report would receive almost

TABLE 5.2

SPECIFICITY OF THE POSITIVE REPORT IN GASTROINTESTINAL CYTOLOGY:
SELECTED SERIES FROM THE LITERATURE

Organ Studied and Authors	Methods	No. of Positive Reports	No. of Proved Cancers	Specificity of Percentage
Esophagus				
Brandborg and Wenger (36)	Saline lavage	48	46	95.8%
Stomach				
Ayre and Oren (10)	Ayre's brush	14	11	78.5%
Brandborg, Taniguchi, and Rubin (34)	"Short" chymotrypsin	107	103	95.4%
Imbriglia, Stein, and Lopusniak (120)	Saline lavage	25	20	80.0%
Klayman et al. (141)	"Long" chymotrypsin	65	60	90.7%
Vilardell (288)	"Mandrel-sonde"	289	280	96.8%
Duodenum				
Dreiling, Nieburgs, and Janowitz (67)	Secretin test	66	54	81.8%
Colon				
Heidenrich (106)	Ayre's brush	40	38	95%

NOTE: Reports using class III or "suspicious" were not included in this table because such reporting makes the analysis impossible.

A less exact way of determining the "specificity" of the positive report, unfortunately, is frequently used by cytologists in reporting their results in the literature— the percentage of patients clinically without cancer who had a positive cytodiagnosis. This quotient usually is

total assurance that he does not have cancer. In other words, the sensitivity index of the negative report has *no clinical value* unless it is accompanied by an almost 100% sensitivity of the positive report, a task certainly impossible in all areas at all times.

Part 3

Material and Results at the University of Chicago:
Discussion and Review of the Literature

6
Washing Cytology of the Esophagus

The tubular shape and relatively easy access of the esophagus make exfoliative cytologic study both easy and accurate. Furthermore, the overwhelming majority of malignant tumors of the esophagus are squamous cell carcinomas, which readily exfoliate diagnostic cells.

Unfortunately, by the time most patients with carcinoma of the esophagus seek medical advice, they already have advanced tumors and the prognosis is very poor. Even the best published results do not exceed a 5% five-year survival rate. Considering the relative ease of the radiologic and endoscopic diagnoses and the high accuracy of cytology, the main problem is not accuracy in diagnosis but rather earlier diagnostic study.

The delay in diagnosis, in our opinion, occurs chiefly because the early symptoms of esophageal carcinoma probably are so minimal as to be disregarded. Dysphagia usually is the first symptom that brings the patient to a physician, but in general it is a manifestation of an advanced tumor. The average delay of three months between the first consultation and the institution of treatment is disturbing but probably not significant in relation to the prognosis (180). Only "presympomatic" diagnosis of esophageal carcinoma, when the lesion remains limited to the walls of the esophagus, offers any hope of better prognosis. Radical surgery cannot be more radical and curative, nor can roentgen therapy be more intense and curative.

However, the low incidence rate of about 2.7 per 100,000 in the United States makes it difficult to institute any large survey or screening programs for asymptomatic carcinoma of the esophagus. Only in countries such as Puerto Rico, Japan and, China, with high incidence rates of upper gastrointestinal cancer, can such programs be considered practical.

For the present, cytology will remain a useful diagnostic technique in patients suspected of esophageal carcinoma, but the outlook for better prognosis is dim. A review of our experience with esophageal cytology in 1965 (210) confirmed the earlier results of Klayman (138) in our laboratory. Since 1965 our experience has been enlarged, and the recent addition of the direct-vision technique (see chap. 8) has further facilitated the procedure.

Material

During the period between April 1955 and December 1968, after exclusion of patients with incomplete followup (less than eighteen months) or inadequate clinical or histologic data, 346 patients were available for the present study, accounting for 382 procedures.

The group of 346 patients comprises 87 with proved malignant tumors and 259 with benign lesions or normal esophagus. This report deals only with the initial examination, but patients with more than one examination, whose initial washing was reported as unsatisfactory but whose repeat examination in the next few days proved to be satisfactory, are listed as positive or negative, as determined in the second study (actually only two patients had positive reports after an initial unsatisfactory test).

The present review includes all patients of the series published in 1965, as stated above (210).

Results

The results are condensed in table 6.1. Of the 87 malignant tumors, 79 were diagnosed correctly, a sensitivity

TABLE 6.1
DIAGNOSTIC ACCURACY OF ESOPHAGEAL CYTOLOGY–
SALINE WASHING METHOD

Lesion	No. of Patients	Positive Cytology	Positive Report Analysis	Negative Cytology
Clinically Benign Lesion or Normal Esophagus	259	4	*Specificity* 95.7%	255
Proved malignant lesions			*Sensitivity*	
Squamous-cell carcinoma	51	47	92.1%	4
Adenocarcinoma, cardia	28	24	85.7%	4
Other [a]	8	8	100.0%	0
Total	87	79	90.8%	8 (9.2%)

NOTE: University of Chicago series, 1955–68; 346 patients.
[a] Gastric carcinoma: 2; tumors of esophagus with histological type not determined: 4; adenocarcinoma of middle third of esophagus: 1; mediastinal mass, adenocarcinoma by biopsy: 1.

of 90.8%. Eight tumors were missed by cytology, an incidence of 9.2% false-negatives in the total series.

Of the 51 squamous cell carcinomas (48 of the esophagus, 2 of the hypopharynx, and 1 of the cardia), 47 were correctly diagnosed, a sensitivity of 92.1%. Of the 28 adenocarcinomas of the cardioesophageal area, 24 were correctly diagnosed, a sensitivity of 85.7%.

The 259 normal or benign lesions of the esophagus were diagnosed correctly in 255 instances; three errors or false-positive diagnoses were in patients with severe ulcerative esophagitis, one additional error was made in a gastric adenomatous polyp located near the cardia. These four instances of false-positive reports represent 4.3% of the total number of positive reports. The specificity of the positive report therefore is 95.7%.

Correlation between the Cytologic and Histopathologic Findings

There are three main histologic categories of squamous cell carcinomas: the well differentiated, the moderately differentiated, and the undifferentiated or anaplastic types. Tumors with definite keratin formation were grouped as differentiated, whereas those without any suggestion of keratin were listed in the anaplastic group.

The differentiated squamous-cell carcinoma always exfoliates cells with sufficient keratinization to be identified easily. The slides, in general, contain large numbers of cells with the criteria set forth for malignant squamous cells. The squamous cancer has a tendency to exfoliate more single cells than clusters, and also to produce malignant pearls and whirls. These cells generally are slightly smaller than the normal squamous cells, but their nuclei are much larger, with an increased nuclear-cytoplasmic ratio. The cytoplasm usually is eosinophilic and keratinized. Less common findings are elongated fiber-like cells and the characteristic tadpole cell.

The undifferentiated squamous-cell carcinoma, on the contrary, never exfoliates cells with distinct keratin formation. Frequently only naked nuclei, clustered and exhibiting the nuclear criteria for malignancy, are observed. If present, the cytoplasm is scanty and basophilic. As we will consider later, a similar cytologic appearance may be observed in some undifferentiated adenocarcinomas of the lower third of the esophagus. This renders the correlation between histopathology and cytology less accurate, and the cytologist should refrain from designating the appearance as other than positive for undifferentiated malignant tumor and compatible with either a squamous or a glandular epithelial origin.

There were twenty-eight cases of adenocarcinoma of the cardioesophageal junction. The typical or well-differentiated adenocarcinoma exfoliates clusters of malignant cells with many cytoplasmic vacuoles, no keratin formation, basophilic cytoplasm, and a substantial overlapping of cells. However, the number of malignant

clusters is not very great, and so all available slides must be carefully screened to establish the diagnosis. As was already indicated, the anaplastic type is difficult to separate from the anaplastic squamous-cell carcinoma. In one case, the histologic picture was of an adenocarcinoma with pronounced squamous metaplasia; the few malignant clusters were of the typical adenocarcinoma type, without signs of squamous metaplasia. A case of polypoid carcinoma with sarcomalike stroma, or so-called carcinosarcoma, exfoliated cells of an undifferentiated type. The morphology of the malignant cells of squamous type is reviewed in detail in part 4.

Comments and Review of the Literature

Cytologic Accuracy. Exfoliative cytology of the saline lavage is remarkably accurate and easily performed. This laboratory was one of the first to call the attention to the high diagnostic accuracy of esophageal cytology (138, 245). Its sensitivity of 90.8% in the presence of a malignant tumor is very favorable. This order of sensitivity has also been reported from other laboratories (table 6.2). Lower figures from some laboratories also have been reported. Johnson and associates (126) reported 69.6%, probably because a Papanicolaou class III reporting was used in 12.2%. Other disappointingly low values of 75% or less have been recorded in the literature, but in general they can be ascribed to less adequate methods of cell collection, including the use of cotton applicators inserted through the esophagoscope or strips of fine-mesh gauze wrapped around gastric tubes or dilators. The incidence of technical failure to secure cytological material is higher with these techniques than with simple lavage.

The value of a negative report has been emphasized previously (219). However, in the presence of an actual tumor, a false-negative report will be issued in approximately 10% of the patients. A negative report is thus not completely reassuring, especially since the gastroenterologist is dealing with a selected group of patients in whom the incidence of malignant tumors is greatly increased.

A totally different approach or appraisal obviously is needed by the clinician screening large groups of asymptomatic people. In the United States, the low incidence of esophageal tumors, the lack of "early" symptoms, and the short clinical history make exfoliative cytology of the esophagus impractical for screening for esophageal cancer in large population groups. The yield of curable cancers almost certainly would be very low. The reported instance of situ carcinoma of the esophagus by Imbriglia and Lopusniak (119), Ushigone, Spjut, and Noon (284), and Koss (151) clearly indicates the sensitivity of the method and its potential use in diagnosing very early lesions. Recently the group of Dr. S. Yamagata in Japan reported two additional cases (304). Unfortunately, for the reasons mentioned the technique is useful only in a selected group of pa-

noma of the esophagus. There probably is insufficient evidence of an increased incidence of esophageal cancer in patients with achalasia to warrant a general screening program. However, because in the instances reported symptoms due to the carcinoma frequently were interpreted as recrudescence of the achalasia, and because of the occasional limitation of radiology in these patients, we include achalasia in this group. The present series includes one patient with Patterson-Plummer-Vinson syndrome followed by a squamous type of esophageal

TABLE 6.2

RESULTS OF ESOPHAGEAL CYTOLOGY: SELECTED SERIES OF THE LITERATURE
(*Proved Malignant Tumors*)

Investigator	Method	Total	Positive	Suspicious or Class III	Negative	Unsatis-factory	Comments
Johnson et al. (126)	Lavage at esopha-goscopy	148	103	18	27	0	
Messelt (181)	Swab at esopha-goscopy	186	141	18	27	Not stated	
Andersen, McDonald, and Olsen (3)	Cotton swab or gauze abrasion at esophagoscopy and with dilators	64	50	0	14	Not stated	Includes 32 cases of carcinoma of the cardia
Hershenson, Lerch, and Hershenson (113)	Gauze abrasion with esophageal dilator	21	16	2	3	0	Includes 8 carcinomas of the cardia—5 unsatisfactory tests (final? diagnosis)
Henning and Witte (110)	"Cell touch probe"	88	70	5	13	0	There is no mention of the benign cases. However, there were 6 false positive reports in the esophagus and stomach series.
Gephart and Graham (84)	Saline lavage	89	67 (73)	7 (7)	14 (8)	1 (1)	Includes 25 cases of carcinoma of the cardia
MacDonald et al. (172)	Ringer's solution lavage	72	63 (68)	5 (0)	6 (4)	0 (0)	Initial test after repeat examination
Klayman (138)	Saline lavage	20	19	0	1	1	University of Chicago series before 1955
Present series	Saline or Ringer's solution lavage	87	79	0	8	2 (Positive on repeat)	University of Chicago series *after* 1955, until December 1968. Includes 28 carcinomas of the cardia.

NOTE: Figures in parentheses indicate final results after repeats of previously negative tests.

tients, mainly those with relatively mild dysphagia or other upper digestive tract symptoms. We also agree with MacDonald and his associates (172) that cytology of the esophagus should be performed at regular intervals of six months or one year in patients predisposed to esophageal cancer: those with lye stricture, Patterson-Plummer-Vinson syndrome, esophageal webs with or without anemia, and previous squamous cell carcinoma of the mouth, in the hope of diagnosing "earlier" carci-

carcinoma and one patient with carcinoma of the left tonsil followed by squamous type of esophageal cancer. The results of a screening project in Puerto Rico, where the incidence of esophageal cancer is very high, reported by Martinez (176), should be of interest.

Errors. Two types of errors are possible: a negative report in the presence of actual malignant tumor—false-negative—and a positive report of malignancy in its

**Material and Results at the
University of Chicago**

absence—false-positive. The problem of false-negatives deserves special mention because increased experience and modifications of the technique should diminish their incidence. The present series contains eight false-negative reports; four tumors of the body of the esophagus (two of which had been previously irradiated) and four in the cardioesophageal junction.

Thus, two circumstances emerge: the absolute need for combined gastric and esophageal washing cytology in any lesion of the cardia and the problem of previously irradiated tumors. In the latter instance, the cytologist should develop experience in the occasionally difficult task of differentiating between irradiation effects and malignant changes. Our false-negative cases occurred in the early years of the laboratory; in recent years there have been no false-negatives for this reason. Actually, the last thirty instances of squamous-cell carcinoma of the esophagus all were correctly diagnosed by exfoliative cytology. Any lesion in the cardioesophageal area should be investigated by both gastric and esophageal cytology to fulfill the prime requisite of recovering cells from above and below the neoplasm. False-negatives numbers 7 and 8 thus can be reclassified as positive, since the gastric cytologic examination was positive. In the chapter on gastric cytology, we will consider the problem of adenocarcinomas of the cardioesophageal junction and the high accuracy of cytology in this type of tumor.

The problem of false-positives is encountered less commonly by the cytologist. But strict criteria of malignant cell identification must be preserved to avoid any undue high incidence, even if this is accomplished at the price of a slightly decreased yield of true positives. In three instances in this series the report of false-positive involved the presence of esophagitis. The cells that misled the cytologist were of the same type described by Gephart and Graham (84), Johnson et al. (126) and Koss (151). It is sufficient to note here that they are now considered to be tissue macrophages or active basal cells. In the series reported by Johnson et al. (126), the false-positives also were due to cellular changes associated with severe ulcerative esophagitis. In Messelt's series also the only false-positive diagnosis was in the presence of chronic esophagitis (181). The preservation of cell adhesion has been considered by Koss (151) as an excellent criterion for the benign nature of the cluster.

In analyzing the cytologic errors, it is important to comment upon the techniques of cell collection used. Saline lavage causes far fewer false-negatives or unsatisfactory examinations. Actually, in our series, there was no unsatisfactory examination in the presence of tumor, and only six of the nine false-negatives were due to failure to recover any malignant cell at all, which could theoretically have been caused by the technique itself. However, we feel that this cause of error can be even smaller if the lesion is brushed under direct vision (see chap. 8).

The safety of the techniques should be noted. The saline washing through a number 16 or 18 french rubber tube is extremely safe and we had no complication of any type. We strongly oppose the blind use of scraping devices, even under fluoroscopic control. Typical of such dangerous methods is "scraping" the esophagus and stomach with aluminum foil tied over the tip of a probe (117). Not surprisingly, a few months after the report of this technique, the same authors reported an instance of hematemesis (184). Raskin's comments on a similar blind or semiblind technique seem appropriate here: "The possibility of perforation or linear rupture in the strictured area or beyond is real and this danger is more acute, I should think, when the stricture is of benign etiology. Once a curette, alligator forceps, cotton ball or bougie enters a strictured area the procedure then for all intent and purpose becomes blind."

Nonmalignant Disease of the Esophagus. Chronic erosive esophagitis has various etiologies, including hiatus hernia, peptic esophagitis, achalasia, and scleroderma. It is an important entity because many cells are exfoliated that can be confused with malignant ones. The histology of chronic esophagitis is a partial or total loss of the surface epithelium and an infiltration of the stroma by chronic inflammatory cells, leading to the formation of erosions and ulcers. Squamous metaplasia of the submucosal glands may occur, and areas of leukoplakia can develop. The cells exfoliated by these lesions resemble active basal cells, "deep cells" as described by Gephart and Graham (84). Their nuclei are large, with some clumping of the chromatin. The cytoplasm is evenly distributed and the cells are not very different from each other. The cells tend to have good adhesion when they occur in groups (210). This point has been used by Koss as an excellent criterion of benignity, as was noted earlier.

The interesting problem of the reaction of the esophageal epithelium to irradiation has been studied by Gephart and Graham (84) and by Goldgraber (92), but it is not yet clear whether the cytologic picture after irradiation could help assess responsiveness to treatment and the prognosis.

Staats, Robinson, and Butterworth (266) made nuclear measurements of oral epithelial cells in twenty-five patients with several clinical types of anemia and in twenty-five individuals without anemia; except that two patients with pernicious anemia had large nuclei, the type of the anemia did not correlate with nuclear size. After one week of therapy, the mean nuclear size of the patients with pernicious anemia had fallen to a level not significantly different from that of the controls. The literature contains numerous references to alterations in nuclear size and in the nuclear-cytoplasmic ratio of oral and esophageal exfoliated cells (177, 185, 204, 307). But these alterations were based on subjective evaluation by the examiner. It should also be kept in mind that the absence of large nuclei does not preclude a diagnosis of pernicious anemia (30).

7
Washing Cytology of the Stomach

Because of the relatively large size of the organ and the digestive capacities of the hydrochloric acid and pepsin in the gastric content, the exfoliative cytology of the stomach is relatively difficult. Meticulous care with washing techniques is important to avoid cellular degeneration that renders cytodiagnosis impossible. Also, various degrees of pyloric obstruction in patients with benign gastric ulcer, carcinoma or stenosing duodenal ulcer cause retention of food and debris, accounting for unsatisfactory examinations in 7% to 10% of the cytologic studies.

In general, the diagnosis of carcinoma of the stomach in symptomatic patients is made after the tumor is advanced. Diagnosis is delayed largely because the patient fails to seek medical attention because of the vague symptoms and partly because of limitations in available diagnostic techniques.

The main diagnostic approach is the roentgenographic examination of the stomach. The technique has a high accuracy potential, but unfortunately faulty roentgen technique is common.

Next in importance is gastroscopy. Until recently, use of this technique was limited because of the lack of competent and trained endoscopists. The recent development of practical and safe fiber-gastroscopes has improved this situation remarkably, and endoscopy now plays a significant role in the diagnosis of gastric lesions.

The role of cytology generally has been limited, and only a few centers have had enough experience and confidence in the method to apply it routinely. The main problem is not difficulty in interpreting the cellular material, but the need for well-trained and meticulous technicians. The simpler direct-vision techniques should improve the situation considerably.

For unknown reasons, attributed by some to diet, there are wide geographic differences in the incidence of gastric carcinoma; at one extreme are countries like Japan, Iceland, Austria, and Chile with very high incidence rates, and at the other extreme countries like the United States with relatively low rates. Interestingly, about two decades ago gastric carcinoma was the most frequent cause of cancer death in the United States. A steady decline, not related to earlier diagnosis or improved treatment, has resulted in the present low death rate.

These geographic differences indicate differing roles for gastric cytology. The rationale and the complexities of mass surveys for gastric carcinoma are discussed in chapter 9. At present, Japan appears to be the only country utilizing such an approach; but the optimal mass-survey method is yet to be designed.

We have given a detailed analysis of our experience with gastric cytology to define its role in the clinical detection of gastric cancer, with special attention to particular problems such as lesions in the cardia, the differential diagnosis of benign gastric ulcer, the ulcer-cancer problem, and the diagnostic examination of the post-operative stomach.

Material

During the period between April 1955 and December 1968, and after the exclusion of patients with incomplete followup (less than 18 mo) or with inadequate clinical or histologic data, 2,575 patients were available for the present study, accounting for 3,291 procedures.

The group of 2,575 patients includes 379 with proved malignancy and 2,196 with benign lesions or negative followup observation. This study deals only with the initial examination. However, patients with more than one study, in whom the initial washing was unsatisfactory but a repeat examination in the next few days proved satisfactory, are listed as positive or negative as determined in the second study. A total of 228 examinations were unsatisfactory, representing 7% of the total number of procedures. In 52 instances, the cytologically unsatisfactory examination could not be repeated; 17 of those were in the malignant group.

The series reported here includes the patients of the series previously reported by Raskin, Kirsner, and Palmer (217) and Taebel, Prolla, and Kirsner (271).

Results

The results are given in table 7.1. Among the 2,196 cases of benign lesions or normal stomach, there were only 5 false-positive reports. In 9 more instances, a positive report was issued and a malignant tumor was found in a neighboring organ (2 in the duodenum, 4 in the pancreas, 2 in the lung, and 1 in the nasopharynx).

Of the 379 malignant lesions, there were 334 adenocarcinomas, 42 malignant lymphomas, 2 leiomyosarcomas, and 1 unclassified malignant tumor. Of the 334 adenocarcinomas, malignant cells were recovered in 259, or 77.5%. Of the 42 malignant lymphomas, 15 were lymphocytic type, 20 were histiocytic type, and 7 were Hodgkin's type. In 27 of the total 42 cases, or 64%, cytology was positive; in 12, cytology was negative; and in 3, cytology was unsatisfactory.

Of the two leiomyosarcomas, one was negative and the other was positive. The unclassified malignant tumor was reported as positive.

Cytohistological Correlation

There were two main types of malignant tumors of the stomach in this series: adenocarcinoma and malignant lymphoma.

Adenocarcinoma

The most typical of all adenocarcinomas of the stomach is the signet ring cell (see part IV for detailed discussion). It is found in almost every case. The second most common cytological presentation consists of clusters of malignant cells of obvious glandular or columnar type; occasionally this will be the only cytological presentation. The least common type is the so-called single-cell pattern (uniformly small and single cells, with scanty cytoplasm).

Lymphoma

The cytological picture of lymphomas of the stomach is described in detail in chapter 15. There was good corre-lation with the histological diagnosis of malignant lymphoma in the positive cases, but not with the histological subtypes (lymphocytic, histiocytic, and Hodgkin's).

Comments and Review of the Literature

Cytological Accuracy

The overall accuracy of the cytologic method, as emphasized previously by this laboratory (217, 271), compares favorably with other techniques of evaluating the upper intestinal tract for malignancy; an accuracy rate similar to ours or higher has been reported by others (e.g., 36, 49, 88, 110, 171, 230, 252, 256).

Only five false-positive reports have been issued, or 1.8% of the total number of positive reports. The high degree of accuracy of the positive report makes it tantamount to a diagnosis of malignancy. The significance of the positive report also is implied by data from most laboratories (table 5.2) and suggests that the diagnostic criteria of the malignant cell originating in the upper intestinal tract are readily identifiable.

However, in additional cases a second type of "false-positive" report was made; true malignant cells were recovered from the gastric washings, but the malignant tumors were situated in organs other than the stomach: the lung, the pancreas, and the esophagus. One of the great advantages of direct-vision cytology is that it elim-

TABLE 7.1

DIAGNOSTIC ACCURACY OF GASTRIC CYTOLOGY WASHING METHOD

Lesion	No. of Patients	Positive Cytology	Positive Report Analysis	Negative Cytology	Unsatisfactory [a]
Clinically benign lesion or normal stomach	2,196 [b]	5	*Specificity* 98.2%	2,147	35
Proved malignant lesions of the stomach:					
Adenocarcinoma	*334*	*259*	*Sensitivity* 77.5%	*61*	*14*
Advanced	(322)	(249)	(77.2%)	(59)	(14)
Superficial ("early")	(12)	(10)	(83.5%)	(2)	—
Malignant lymphoma	*42*	*27*	64.0%	*12*	*3*
Lymphocytic	(15)	(11)	—	(4)	—
Histiocytic	(20)	(12)	—	(6)	(2)
Hodgkin's	(7)	(4)	—	(2)	(1)
Leiomyosarcoma	*2*	*1*	—	*1*	—
Other	*1*	*1*	—	*0*	—
Total	379	288	76.6%	74 (19%)	17 (44%)

NOTE: University of Chicago Series, 1955–68; 2,575 patients
[a] Not repeated within 2 wk.
[b] In 9 patients a positive cytology was obtained, and the malignant tumor was found elsewhere: 2 in duodenum, 4 in pancreas, 2 in lung, 1 in nasopharynx.

**Material and Results at the
University of Chicago**

inates these errors, the material being collected directly from the gastric lesion.

In this series, false-negative reports were issued in 61 cases of proved adenocarcinoma, in 12 cases of malignant lymphoma, and in 1 leiomyosarcoma. A review of this material indicates that of the 61 adenocarcinomas, only 3 had suspicious cells designated as negative. Three other cases, upon review, demonstrated malignant cells, and these are classified as a "reader's error." Of the remaining 55 false-negative cases of adenocarcinoma, the false-negative report seemed to be primarily a function of inability to obtain exfoliated malignant cells.

Of the 12 false-negative lymphomas, 8 had normal preparations with good exfoliation, and 4 contained atypical gastric epithelial cells. Extensive retrospective review of the slides of these cases failed to reveal any instance of "reader's error" and indicated that screening, although difficult, was accurate and that the error was in the sampling. The reason for the lower accuracy rate is complex and includes the probability that the malignant lymphoma occasionally may be located entirely within the submucosa or that the "lymphoma cells" may be rapidly destroyed in the gastric content. Regardless, the present results indicate that exfoliative cytology has not been a highly accurate method for diagnosing malignant lymphoma of the stomach (208) (table 7.2), an experience shared by others.

However, as is noted in table 7.3, the addition of cytology improved the diagnosis of malignant lymphoma. In 12 of the 40 patients so examined, the roentgenographic diagnosis was normal stomach in 9 patients and benign ulcer in 3. Cytology was positive for malignant lymphoma in 6 of these patients. Furthermore, in 15 cases in which the roentgenographic diagnosis was gastric carcinoma, cytology was positive for malignant lymphoma in 10 instances.

Similarly, cytology "corrected" the negative endoscopic diagnosis in 3 instances, and of the 16 patients in which the diagnosis was carcinoma, cytology was positive for lymphoma in 9.

Anatomical Location of the Tumor

Among the 281 malignant lesions with available X-ray reports, the radiologist was able to detect an abnormality in all but 14, a detection rate of 95%. The radiologist was

TABLE 7.2

DIAGNOSTIC CYTOLOGY IN MALIGNANT LYMPHOMAS INVOLVING THE STOMACH

Author	Method	No. of Patients	Positive Cytology	Detection Rate [a] (%)	Comments
MacDonald et al. (171)	Chymotrypsin	4	4	100	In 9 patients cytology was repeated because of large lymphocytes, and in 1 additional patient cytology was falsely positive for lymphoma.
Seybolt, Papanicolaou, and Cooper (257)	Abrasive balloon	16	4	37.5	In 5 additional patients, cytology was class III
Vilardell (288)	"Mandrel tube" (abrasion and washing)	7	3	42.8	
Umiker et al. (282)	Chymotrypsin lavage	4	2	50	In the other 2 patients, cytology was "suspicious"
Shida and Tsuda (260)	Several methods (abrasive, lavage, direct vision)	5 (?)	5	—	Total number of patients with lymphoma not stated; detection rate could not be calculated.
Yoshii et al. (306)	Imprint cytology under direct vision	4	4	100	Biopsy was positive in only 2 of the 4 patients.
Present series	a) Saline or Ringer's solution lavage	42	27	64	Including all cases previously reported (139,271)
	b) Direct-vision brushing	4	3	75	Cases seen between August 1968 and 30 June 1970.
	c) Total experience	46	30	65.2	

[a] It is obvious that in most series the number of cases is too small for accurate detection rates to be calculated, and the reported cases may represent selected cases only.

able to render an opinion that the lesion was malignant in 72%. In 1960, Strandjord, Moseley, and Schweinefus from our department of radiology, reviewed the accuracy of the roentgenographic method in the diagnosis of gastric carcinoma. Their series included some of the patients in the present study. It is interesting that the radiologist was able to detect some abnormality in 95% of the examinations, and a correct diagnosis of cancer was made in 85% of the cases.

TABLE 7.3

CYTOLOGICAL, RADIOLOGICAL, AND ENDOSCOPICAL CORRELATIONS
IN 42 CASES OF MALIGNANT LYMPHOMA OF THE STOMACH

| Diagnosis | Cytology | | | Total |
	Positive for Lymphoma	Negative	Unsatis-factory	
X rays				
1. Negative	5	4	—	9 ⎫ 12/40
2. Benign gastric ulcer	1	2	—	3 ⎬
3. Carcinoma	10	5	—	15 ⎫
4. Carcinoma × lymphoma	5	—	2	7 ⎬ 28/40
5. Lymphoma	5	1	—	6 ⎭
Endoscopy				
1. Negative	3	3	—	6 ⎫ 7/32
2. Benign gastric ulcer	—	1	—	1 ⎬
3. Carcinoma	9	6	1	16 ⎫
4. Carcinoma × lymphoma	1	1	—	2 ⎬ 25/32
5. Lymphoma	5	1	1	7 ⎭

SOURCE: Prolla, Kobayashi, and Kirsner (208).

Probably in many instances the X ray was so unequivocal that a definitive surgical therapeutic approach could be initiated solely on the radiographic impression. But when the malignancy involves the cardia or the antrum, the X-ray examination becomes less reliable, and supplemental diagnostic methods are essential for a definitive diagnosis. This is particularly true in evaluating the operated stomach for the possible recurrence of malignancy or for the occasional development of a tumor on a stomach previously operated for a benign condition. The accuracy of exfoliative cytology, therefore, was evaluated in each of these situations. The depth of invasion by carcinoma in the gastric wall is also an important prognostic factor, and the group of superficial (invasion limited to mucosa or submucosa) gastric carcinomas was evaluated.

Malignant Lesions of the Cardia

The malignant tumor was placed in this group if it extended across the cardioesophageal junction. Seventy-two malignancies involved this area: 71 adenocarcinomas and 1 reticulum cell sarcoma. The X ray was diagnostic of malignancy in 80%, reported the lesion as benign in 8%, and could not differentiate in 12%. The cytology report was positive in 93% of these patients (table 7.4).

The accuracy of X ray in this category is higher than that reported in other series (210); yet the still relatively large percentage of inconclusive or incorrect reports indicates the need for a comprehensive approach to patients suspected of having lesions involving the cardia. The difficulty of adequate endoscopic examination of this region of the stomach has been described (24, 210). Because of the high accuracy of exfoliative cytology, this method is of particular diagnostic value.

Significantly, of the 72 malignancies, 24 were studied by the esophageal lavage technique and 48 by esophageal or gastric lavage or both. It has been almost routine in this laboratory to perform both procedures when the cardia is suspect on the basis of clinical complaints or, more often, when the X ray has indicated an abnormality in that area. As is seen in table 7.4, the detection rate varies considerably in the reported series. The lavage method appears to give the best yield, but there are exceptions. Also, many series do not have complete information about the number of unsatisfactory examinations, and others include the "suspicious" category in their reports.

Malignant Lesions of the Antrum

Eighty-three malignancies of the antrum were evaluated cytologically: 78 adenocarcinomas and 5 malignant lymphomas. Among these 83, the X ray was diagnostic of malignancy in 65%, reported the abnormality as benign in 10%, and was inconclusive in 25%. Cytology was positive in 68, or 81%.

In a series of 1,866 patients reported previously (271), an antral abnormality was the reason given for the cytological examination in 440. Such an abnormality, therefore, was the most common indication for the examination and probably reflects the frequent involvement of the antrum with gastritis, ulceration, scarring, and adenocarcinoma, all of which may produce altera-

**Material and Results at the
University of Chicago**

TABLE 7.4

DETECTION RATE OF DIAGNOSTIC CYTOLOGY IN MALIGNANT LESIONS OF THE CARDIA

Author	Method	No. of Patients	Positive Cytology	Detection Rate (%)	Comments
Gephart and Graham (84)	Saline washings	25	16	64	In 4 additional patients a "suspicious" report was issued
Messelt (181)	Cotton swabs at esophagoscopy (under general anesthesia	43	13	30	Ten additional "suspicious" reports were issued
Vilardell (288)	"Mandrel tube" (abrasion and washing)	89	83	93.2	Includes some cases of the gastric fundus
Schickendantz et al. (253)	Ayre's brush	26	19	73	Unsatisfactory cases were excluded (numbers not stated); in 4 additional cases cytology was "suspicious"
Andersen, McDonald, and Olsen (3)	Smears from dilators or esophagoscope	32	26	81.2	No statement about number of unsatisfactory cases
Present series	Esophageal and/or gastric saline or Ringer's solution lavage	72	67	93.0	In 2 patients, esophageal lavage was negative but gastric lavage was positive
Present series	Direct-vision brushing	10	8	80	Relatively small series

tions in the roentgen appearance which are virtually impossible to differentiate. The accuracy of the cytological examination in evaluating the antrum deserves more emphasis.

Gastric Ulcer (Table 7.5)

A review of our material revealed 476 benign gastric ulcers and 65 malignant gastric ulcers studied by washing cytology (211, 212). The malignant gastric ulcer was placed in this group if the pathological description coincided with the type described by Stout (268) as a penetrating adenocarcinoma with central ulceration or a Borrmann's type II tumor. There were 61 such malignant ulcers and 4 ulcerative malignant lymphomas, histiocytic type, included because of the similar macroscopical appearance.

Attesting to the diagnostic difficulty with this type of ulcer, roentgenography was reported as malignant ulcer in 32 patients (49%), as benign ulcer in 18 patients (23%), and as undetermined in 15 patients (28%) on the initial examinations. A positive cytodiagnosis was obtained in 46 of the 65 patients (71%), as is seen in table 7.5. In 20 of the 33 patients in whom the roentgenographic diagnosis was inconclusive or indicated benign gastric ulcer, cytology was correctly positive, a finding of significant supplemental clinical value.

Unfortunately, the detection rate of the cytological

study is somewhat lower with the ulcer-cancer type of lesion than with gastric carcinoma in general, an observation also made by others (153, 287, 301). In almost every report in which we could separate the "ulcer-cancers," the detection rate approximated 70%. The reasons for this lower diagnostic accuracy are not clear, but they may be related to the necrosis accompanying ulceration, which may render the malignant cells too degenerated for accurate identification (287).

In the very small group of malignant ulcers studied by the brushing method (see chap. 8), a positive cytodiagnosis was obtained in all 3 patients—too small a group for analysis. However, in the Japanese experience (118, 132, 133, 144), direct-vision cytology of small ulcerated gastric carcinomas—especially of the "early" type—is highly accurate, usually exceeding 90%.

In our opinion, every gastric ulcer should be evaluated by cytology in addition to roentgenography and endoscopy. If available, the direct-vision method yields better results and should be employed. Concomitant gastric biopsy under direct vision will produce a combined accuracy of nearly 100% (148). The most important role of cytology is to detect those cases of gastric carcinoma missed by roentgenography and endoscopy. The value of the negative cytology result is difficult to evaluate, and in the case of saline washings cytology does not exclude malignancy with enough certainty to

TABLE 7.5

DETECTION RATE OF DIAGNOSTIC CYTOLOGY IN MALIGNANT GASTRIC ULCER:
COMMENTS ON THE SPECIFICITY OF THE POSITIVE REPORT

Author	Method	No. of Patients	Positive Cytology	Detection Rate (%)	Comments
Witte and Bressell (301)	"Cell touch probe"	7	2 (actually only "suspicious")	(Series too small)	In 4 out of 48 (8%) of benign ulcers, cytology was suspicious of cancer
Umiker et al. (282)	Chymotrypsin lavage	14	7	50	In 5 additional patients, cytology was "suspicious" of cancer
Vilardell (288)	"Mandrel tube" (abrasion plus washings)	59	45	76.2	The authors reported 5 false-positive reports in patients with peptic ulcer (total number not stated)
Kurokawa et al. (153)	Gastric abrasive balloon	73	54	74.0	Borrmann type II; in 168 cases of benign gastric ulcer, there were 10 false-positive and 5 Class III cytology reports
Present series	Ringer's solution or saline lavage	65	46	70.7	One false-positive cytology was found among 476 benign gastric ulcers seen during the same period

warrant conservative medical treatment if the other diagnostic procedures indicate a malignancy.

The cytopathologist must be aware of the atypical cells associated with benign gastric ulcer. In reviewing our material (211, 212), and as is discussed in chapter 14, several degrees of cellular atypia are observed. Other authors also have made false-positive reports in the presence of benign gastric ulcer (table 7.5). The experience of Witte (298) and Witte and Bressel (301) is particularly pertinent because they described similar cellular atypias.

The Use of Gastric Cytology in the Operated Stomach

The previously operated stomach offers considerable diagnostic difficulties, especially in its radiological appearance. The most difficult question always is how to differentiate between surgical scarring and deformity from malignant tumor (local recurrence or, more rarely, de novo tumor formation).

In our experience, diagnostic cytology can be very helpful in evaluating patients who have undergone gastric surgery. For convenience of analysis, our 102 patients are divided into four groups (table 7.6).

Group 1. Evaluation of local recurrence of malignant tumors, with proved tumor recurrence: 26 patients

Group 2. Evaluation of local recurrence of malignant

TABLE 7.6

DIAGNOSTIC CYTOLOGY IN THE OPERATED STOMACH

Groups of Patients	No. of Patients	Positive Cytology	Negative Cytology	Comments
Group 1. Proved recurrent tumors	26	25	1	Very high detection rate of recurrent tumors
Group 2. No recurrent tumor	16	—	16	No false-positives
Group 3.[a] Late appearance of carcinoma in operated stomach (for benign diseases)	7	5	2	See Kobayashi, Prolla, and Kirsner (146) for detailed report of such cases
Group 4. Postoperative stomach (for benign disease)	52	—	52	No false positives

NOTE: University of Chicago series.
[a] In one patient, cytology was done by the direct-vision method. In all other cases, the washing method was used.

tumors, with proved lack of recurrences: 16 patients

Group 3. Late development of gastric carcinoma in stomach operated for benign conditions: 7 patients

**Material and Results at the
University of Chicago**

Group 4. Evaluation of previously operated stomachs
for benign conditions, with negative long-term
followup: 52 patients

Special technical difficulties may be encountered during the cytological examination of these patients; a small gastric remnant and a wide stoma hamper full recovery of the washing solution; and food retention is frequent in the presence of tumor or other pathological conditions of the stoma. Additional care is needed to surmount these difficulties. Using smaller volumes of washing fluid (50 ml instead of the usual 100 ml), the left side recumbent position and slight elevation of the foot of the bed (Trendlenburg position), previous aspiration and saline lavage of the pouch in the presence of food retention, all help improve the quality of the cytological examination. The recent availability of direct-vision cytology also has facilitated cell collection in these patients.

Group 1. Proved Recurrent Tumors

This survey included 26 recurrent adenocarcinomas of the stomach. The cytological examination for possible recurrence was performed from three months to seven years after the initial resection. Two cases were examined thirteen and seventeen years after resection respectively and, although included in this group, the "recurrent" tumors probably represent entirely new lesions. Surgical exploration or autopsy was performed in 22 cases, with confirmation of recurrence in the gastric remnant or at the anastomosis. The remaining 4 patients died within several months of the cytological study with findings of tumor recurrence.

As noted in table 7.6, cytology was positive in 25 instances (96%). The clinical value of cytology is best appreciated when the results of X ray and endoscopy are taken into consideration. X rays were performed in 23 cases; a definite diagnosis of local recurrence was achieved in only 10 instances. Cytology was positive in 12 of the 13 cases with inconclusive (7 cases) or negative (6 cases) radiological findings. Endoscopy was performed in only 12 instances; in 9 a positive identification of local recurrence was achieved. In the 3 negative cases, cytology was positive in all. Of the entire series of 26 cases, only 1 was missed by radiology and cytology and had no endoscopic examination.

The development of recurrent tumor probably is related to the high incidence of tumor found microscopically at the resection line—as high as 40%. Less frequent is the development of a second gastric adenocarcinoma. In the series reported by Fridman (75), recurrent tumor was present in the gastric remnant in 60% of cases; many were detected two to three years after the initial surgery. Ordinarily, demonstrating recurrence is considered to be only of prognostic interest because of the high incidence of concurrent metastases. That this may not always be the situation is implied by the findings of Stout (268): of 6 patients with recurrent tumor, only 3 had evidence of metastases. In 74 patients with recurrence described by Fridman (75), 12 were found at autopsy to have only local recurrence without metastases. In our series, of the 15 cases explored or autopsied, 12 were found to have metastases; of the remaining 3, 2 had inoperable masses at the anastomosis. In the third case, the residual gastric remnant was resected, but the patient died of widespread carcinoma seven months after operation. Thus, the incidence of concurrent metastases undoubtedly is high, although the metastases may have developed from the recurrent tumor. The ability to detect early recurrence may be an important factor, then, in reducing the frequency of concurrent metastases.

X ray is the diagnostic procedure most commonly employed for this purpose, even though the postoperative state is difficult to evaluate. Early postoperative radiologic examination facilitates later comparison. Of the 26 patients in this series with recurrent tumors, 6 had at least one X ray between surgery and the time when cytology for possible recurrence was obtained, at which time another X ray was taken. Even with the earlier radiologic studies, in only 1 case could the radiologist diagnose recurrence; in the remaining 5 he reported no recurrence or was unable to differentiate scarring from recurrence.

The accurate results of the cytological study suggest that this procedure is a useful complementary method of studying the patient with previous gastric resection for adenocarcinoma and perhaps, if repeated regularly, may allow earlier detection of recurrences and thus improve the selection of patients for further surgery.

Group 2. Negative Followup for Recurrent Tumor

In 16 patients the clinical course (five-year survival), surgical exploration, or autopsy gave evidence of no recurrent tumor. In all, cytology was reported as negative for malignant cells. The radiological examinations in these patients were reported as normal postoperative stomach, without evidence of local recurrence, in 11 patients; as revealing recurrent tumor in 2; and as inconclusive in 3. Gastroscopy was performed in 8 patients; in 6 the report was normal postoperative stump without recurrent tumor, and in 2 patients there was local recurrence.

The role of the negative cytology in evaluating these patients is difficult to assess. In patients with both negative X rays and endoscopy, it is reassuring further evidence of the absence of local recurrence and should lead only to followup studies every six months, until a five-year survival period is achieved. In patients with radiological or endoscopical evidence of recurrence, the negative cytological result must be questioned, at least until confirmed. The first approach should be a repeat study. If this examination also is negative, two alternatives remain: wait and repeat all studies in three to six months, or explore the patient (if there are no signs of distant spread). We favor the latter alternative.

Group 3. Late Development of Carcinoma after Operation for Benign Conditions (146)

Table 7.7 lists 7 cases of carcinoma in the gastric remnant operated upon originally for benign gastroduodenal disease, seen at the Gastroenterology Section at the University of Chicago since 1958. The indication for op-

eration had been duodenal ulcer in 5 cases, pyloric ulcer in 1 case, and "hyperacidity" in 1 patient. The operations performed were gastroenterostomy with partial gastric resection (Billroth type II) in 2 cases, Billroth I operation in 1, and gastoenterostomy without gastric resection in 4. The anastomotic area was involved by the carcinoma in all 7 cases. In 4 patients, the main tumor was at the anastomosis. In cases 4 and 5, there was extensive carcinomatous infiltration in the anastomotic area. In case 3, the main tumor was present in the antrum, extending to involve the anastomosis.

All patients were diagnosed correctly by at least one method. Both gastroscopy and cytology established the diagnosis in 5 cases. X-ray examination of the upper gastrointestinal tract, however, was reported as suspicious in only 2 instances; a marginal ulcer was suspected in 3 instances, and X rays were reported as normal in 2 cases. Survival was very poor and all patients except case 7, which is under current followup, died within one year after the second operation. Only in this last patient was direct-vision biopsy by the Olympus Gastro-Fiberscope used, and this procedure correctly demonstrated the adenocarcinoma.

Gastroscopy and cytology were more useful diagnostic procedures in this group than radiology. The literature contains numerous references to the limitations of X ray in the diagnosis of postresection carcinoma, the

TABLE 7.7

Late Development of Adenocarcinoma in Postoperative Stomach
(*Case Summaries*)

Case No.	Original Diagnosis	Original Operation	Age (Years)	Interval [a] (Years)	Location of Tumor	Diagnosis of Carcinoma			Survival after Diagnosis (Years)
						Radiology	Gastroscopy	Cytology	
1	D.U.[b]	G.E.[b]	43	14	Stoma	Incorrect	Incorrect	Positive	Less than 1
2	D.U.	Billroth I	60	35	Stoma	Incorrect	Correct	Positive	Less than 1
3	D.U.	G.E.	70	15	Stoma + antrum	Incorrect	Correct	Negative	Less than 1
4	D.U.	G.E.	50	22	Stoma + antrum	Incorrect	Correct	Negative	Less than 1
5	D.U.	Billroth II	64	38	Stoma + diffuse	Correct	Correct	Positive	Less than 1
6	G.U.[b]	G.E.	60	23	Stoma	Correct	Correct	Positive	Less than 1
7	"Hyperacidity"	Billroth II	66	14	Stoma	Incorrect	Correct	Positive (Biopsy positive)	Followup

Source: Kobayashi, Prolla, and Kirsner (146).
[a] Interval between primary operation and diagnosis of carcinoma.
[b] D.U., duodenal ulcer; G.U., gastric ulcer; G.E., gastroenterostomy.

**Material and Results at the
University of Chicago**

diagnostic accuracy varying from 20% to 50%. Most of the interpretations by X ray were marginal ulcer or recurrent ulcer with complication (7, 17, 19, 50, 53, 87, 196). However, the double-contrast roentgen method has been emphasized as helpful in the early diagnosis of carcinoma and in differentiating such a lesion from a marginal ulcer. On the other hand, Lecomte et al. (158) reported a correct X ray diagnosis in 22 of 23 cases, and Gerstenberg et al. (85) commented that radiology provides the most convincing evidence of gastric stump carcinoma. The result seems to depend upon each radiologist's technique and interpretation.

Using gastroscopy, Berkowitz, Cooney, and Bralow (17) succeeded in establishing a correct diagnosis in 3 of 5 cases and ascribed the failures to the absence of an adequate pouch, preventing full distention, so that a large lesion on the greater curvature and involving the posterior wall might be overlooked. In our experience, endoscopic observation of the postoperative stomach is adequately performed by the modern fiberoptic esophagoscope with a forward view of the field. A few reports concerning cytological diagnosis are available. Gibbs (87, 88) has noted that cytology probably is the only method now available whereby a precise preoperative diagnosis of malignancy can be obtained in patients who previously have undergone gastric surgery. Our results, with cytology detecting 5 of 7 cases, support Gibbs's opinion.

Group 4. Stomachs Operated upon for Benign Lesions with Negative Followup

This group served as a control for the specificity and accuracy of the method. A total of 52 patients whose stomachs had been previously operated upon (with some degree of gastric resection) were studied, all with negative cytology reports. In 3 patients the endoscopy report raised the possibility of tumor, and in 2 other patients the X-ray studies suggested this possibility. Subsequent studies and followup, as well as the cytologic examinations, were negative.

Superficial (Early) Gastric Carcinoma

In 12 of the 334 patients with gastric adenocarcinoma (table 7.1), the lesion was confined to the mucosa or submucosa. This type of lesion is frequently referred to in the literature as superficial or "early" gastric carcinoma (102, 149, 203, 207, 267).

As will be discussed in chapter 8, 3 additional cases

were seen after 1968 and studied by direct-vision brushing cytology, increasing our total experience with superficial gastric carcinoma to 15 patients. A positive cytodiagnosis was made in 13 instances (86.6%). Cytologically, the superficial and the frankly invasive carcinomas did not differ from each other.

This group of gastric carcinomas is very important because of its excellent prognosis after surgery. The Japanese have the largest experience with this type of tumor and reported a 92.5% five-year survival rate (105), as we discussed in a recent review of this problem (207). The Japanese are using the direct-vision cytology techniques with great accuracy, reporting 90% to 98% detection rates.

Outside Japan, the experience of Schade (252) in England also is noteworthy. Observing a group of patients with chronic atrophic gastritis, he has been able to detect 60 cases of superficial gastric carcinomas, some of them microscopic in size.

Gastric Cytology in Benign Lesions Other Than Peptic Ulcer

We commented earlier in this chapter on the problems of cytology in gastric ulcers. Frequently other benign lesions are clinical problems, and cytology is indicated whenever there is suspicion of malignancy.

Adenomatous Polyps

In the present series, 37 cases with adenomatous polyps of the stomach were studied by cytology. One false-positive cytology was seen in this group. Except for this case, no prominent cellular atypias were noted in the material. In some instances, increased numbers of goblet cells were seen, probably owing to associated chronic gastritis. Also, an increased degree of polymorphonuclear invasion of columnar cells was seen. This finding, in the experience of Gibbs (88), which we confirmed, is indicative of both superficial and chronic gastritis. No morphological detail was seen that could identify the cases of adenomatous polyps from other benign lesions.

Chronic Gastritis and Atrophic Gastritis

The clinical importance of these lesions resides in their premalignant potential, according to many investigators. As is noted elsewhere, the experience of Schade (250–52) in England is particularly important; he has been able to detect a significant number of superficial gastric carcinomas in a preclinical stage, following patients with chronic gastritis by cytological examinations. In chapter 14, we present the several types of cells seen in chronic gastritis.

Interestingly, in 1964 Boon et al. (31) failed to show the value of cytology in an attempt at presymptomatic diagnosis of gastric carcinoma in 282 patients with pernicious anemia; only 2 carcinomas were detected, both inoperable. MacDonald et al. (170), also in 1964, reached similar conclusions, examining 500 patients with pernicious anemia or hypochlorhydria.

Gastric Syphilis

As we noted elsewhere (209), this rare lesion has a characteristic cytological picture, similar to that of other chronic inflammatory lesions such as tuberculosis, sarcoidosis, or Crohn's disease (15, 54, 134, 191, 216, 270). The difficulties in interpretation have caused some false-positive cytodiagnoses (134, 191) in gastric syphilis as well as in similar inflammatory conditions (15, 270). The cellular characteristics of these lesions are described in chapter 14.

Reactive Lymphoreticular Hyperplasia (Pseudolymphoma)

This unusual lesion is important because of its frequent confusion with the malignant true lymphoma. As is explained in chapter 15, the cytological diagnosis is difficult, but possible (147).

8

Direct-Vision Cytology of the Esophagus and Stomach

The successful development of fiberoptic endoscopes has made possible more widespread use of endoscopy in the evaluation of lesions of the upper gastrointestinal tract. More recently, the Japanese have designed fiberoptic endoscopes incorporating a mechanism whereby lesions may be brushed or washed to exfoliate cells for cytodiagnosis or biopsies may be made under direct observation. In their experience (130–33, 280), confirmed by our own, these techniques are both easy and accurate; the combined use of biopsy and cytology gives an accuracy rate of nearly 100%. The method of direct-vision cytology also is being introduced in Europe, as is attested by some preliminary small series (60, 296, 300). As will be seen later in this chapter, there are several advantages to the direct-vision brushing technique, and the method has progressively replaced "blind" washing in our laboratory. At present, the latter method is used only when endoscopy is contraindicated.

The abundant cellular material obtained by the brushing technique has facilitated the study of two additional staining methods—the polychromic stain of Shorr, and Bertalanffy's Acridine-Orange fluorescence miscroscopy. These two methods are important for their potential value in mass surveys, because of the small amount of time needed for fixation and staining (see chap. 4 for technical details). The technique of direct-vision brushing is described in chapter 3, "Methods of Cell Collection." A preliminary report of our data has been published (145), including data from August 1968 to 30 September 1969.

Material and Results

Papanicolaou Staining

This method was performed in 240 patients (49 with cancer and 191 with other processes) during the period August 1968 to 30 June 1970. The diagnostic accuracy was 89.7% in the cancer cases. A false-positive diagnosis was made in three instances (table 8.1). Table 8.2 shows the results in various types of tumors.

In our series, three instances of early (superficial) gastric carcinoma, in which carcinomatous invasion is confined to the mucosa or submucosa, were detected by this method. Roentgenographic examination of the stomach was normal in two instances and revealed a benign gastric ulcer in the third.

Acridine-Orange Technique

Table 8.4 presents the results in 185 patients (cases up to 30 June 1970). A positive result was obtained in 24 out of 34 patients with malignant tumors, and one false-positive result was issued. (Since this approach was experimental, no report was sent to the attending physician.)

Shorr Technique (Table 8.5)

This approach was utilized in 140 patients up to 30 June 1970. A positive result was obtained in 18 of the 25

TABLE 8.1

DIAGNOSTIC ACCURACY OF GASTROESOPHAGEAL BRUSHING CYTOLOGY UNDER DIRECT VISION

	No. of Patients	Cytology Positive	Cytology Negative	Positive Percentage (± S.E.)
Cancer	49	44	5	89.7 ± 4.3%
Not cancer	191	3	188	1.5 ± 0.85%

NOTE: University of Chicago series, August 1968 to June 1970; 240 patients. The Papanicolaou staining method was used.

patients with malignant tumors, and no false-positive report was issued.

Discussion

Various cytological methods under direct vision with a fiberoptic instrument have been introduced—lavage by Kasugai in 1964 (131); brushing by Kameya et al. in 1964 (130); and suction by Kidokoro et al. in 1965 (135)—to achieve better diagnostic results in gastric carcinoma.

Since then, many reports have been published: lavage (77, 121, 144), aspiration by a polyethylene tube (136), scraping with a sponge ball (104), and brushing with a nylon brush (118, 279). Diagnostic accuracy has been excellent, ranging from 90% to 98%, comparable with our study. In the last report from the group of Kasugai (144), the procedure was performed in 375 patients with proved gastric cancer, and of these 363, or 96.8%, were positive. Sixty-four cases had early gastric cancer, with positive cytology results in 62 (97%).

However, one major limitation of the otherwise excellent contribution of the Japanese workers might be in the extent and thoroughness of their followup of negative cytology reports. Only after a large series with such outstanding accuracy values is properly validated by careful followup, with comparisons and conclusions, can the data be regarded as authoritative. Also, some of their examples of "early" gastric carcinoma, especially of the elevated or polypoid types, judging from the available illustrations, probably would not be diagnosed as carcinomas by most American pathologists. A more thorough discussion of this subject is needed. Fortunately, such debatable cases usually represent a small percentage of their series.

Anatomical and Histological Types of Malignant Tumors

The 49 malignant tumors (table 8.2) were subdivided into four subgroups. There were 9 squamous-cell carcinomas of the esophagus; all were positive by cytology.

TABLE 8.2

RESULTS OF DIRECT-VISION BRUSHING CYTOLOGY
IN GASTROESOPHAGEAL MALIGNANT TUMORS

	No. of Patients	Positive Cytology	Negative Cytology
Squamous-cell carcinoma, esophagus	9	9	0
Adenocarcinoma, cardia	10	8	2
Adenocarcinoma, stomach	26	24	2
Malignant lymphoma, stomach	4	3	1
Totals	49	44	5

NOTE: The Papanicolaou staining method was used.

Although this is an impressive detection rate, 100%, the series is yet too small for valid statistical conclusions.

There were 10 adenocarcinomas of the cardia, of which 8 were positive. The cardia remains a difficult area for endoscopic methods, and washing cytology should be performed in every negative case.

There were 26 adenocarcinomas of the stomach, 24 of which were positive. The detection rate of 92.3% for gastric adenocarcinoma is significantly better than the 77.5% rate of saline washings.

In 3 patients, the adenocarcinoma was of the superficial ("early") type. Cytology was positive in all three instances. The first case seen has been reported in detail (150).

There were only 4 malignant lymphomas of the stomach, of which 3 were positive. As is indicated else-

where, we hope that in a larger series direct-vision cytology will prove more accurate than the 64% diagnostic rate of saline washings.

Advantages

The "brushing" technique has several advantages (145, 296):

a) Brushing is performed simultaneously with endoscopy, obviating a second procedure for both physician and patient. A biopsy is routinely done immediately after brushing.

b) Cells are obtained easily and selectively directly from the lesion under direct vision.

c) The time needed for the cytologic procedure itself is very short, since brushing is done selectively and smears are prepared immediately without need for centrifugation or other processing.

d) There is no need for cytotechnologists to be specially trained in the cumbersome cell-collection methods of blind lavages.

e) The smears obtained are rich in well-preserved cells from the lesion itself and the very light and clean background makes screening easy and quick.

f) The procedure is very safe. We have had no complications.

False-Negative Cytology

Two instances of adenocarcinoma of the cardia were negative by cytology. In both, the esophagofiberscope was used, and the instrument could not be advanced into the stomach. Only the most proximal portions of the tumor were seen, and the brushings collected only mucus and cellular debris, too degenerated for cytological evaluation. In one case careful review of the slides, after the definitive diagnosis was established, revealed a few scattered malignant cells overlooked by the screeners.

Two false-negative diagnoses by cytology were encountered in patients with adenocarcinoma of the stomach. In the first case, multiple gastric ulcers were present in the antrum. The X-ray diagnosis was benign gastric ulcers. Gastroscopy revealed multiple benign-appearing ulcers in the antrum, except for one irregular ulcer with surrounding erythema and edema, and a somewhat dirty base. However, the final impression was that they were most likely multiple benign ulcers. Two brushings were taken from the vicinity of the irregular ulcer and two

**Material and Results at the
University of Chicago**

biopsies were taken from the edges. Cytology was negative, but the biopsy was positive for malignancy. Histology of the resected specimen revealed carcinoma cells only in the submucosal layer of the mucosa adjacent to the ulcers, which appeared intact. This was a case of Borrmann type IV carcinoma (predominantly submucosal), which sometimes is slow to yield malignant cells even by the direct-vision method (305). Biopsy successfully established the correct diagnosis on this patient.

In the other case, a large fungating carcinoma was easily brushed, but again only necrotic debris was collected. Biopsy was unequivocally positive.

One case of malignant lymphoma, histiocytic type, was negative. Only epithelial cells and leukocytes were seen in the smears. This is not surprising, because of the mainly submucosal location of the tumor.

False-Positive Cytology

Three false-positive cytologies were reported: two cases with benign gastric ulcers proved by surgery, and one instance with recurrent esophagitis. In the first case, with a single gastric ulcer at the gastric angulus, a number of abnormal mitoses were seen in groups of cells exfoliated in two different examinations. For this reason, biopsy was indicated and five pieces were taken from the margins of the ulcer, all of which were negative for malignancy. Eventually the patient was operated upon, and histology revealed a benign gastric ulcer. The multiple mitoses were attributed to an actively regenerating epithelium and were misinterpreted as indicative of malignancy. Another patient with multiple gastric ulcers on the greater curvature of the antrum, with slight suspicion of early gastric carcinoma as interpreted by endoscopy, was misdiagnosed cytologically for the same reason. It should be pointed out that other malignant features were not recognized in the cytological specimen in these cases, and the presence of mitoses only should not be overemphasized diagnostically.

In the one patient with a false-positive esophageal cytology, esophagoscopy revealed a mass on the anterior aspect and a widely eroded area with active bleeding on the posterior wall at the cardioesophageal junction. The endoscopic impression was carcinoma. Cytology was performed three times; the first two examinations were positive and the last one was negative. The positive cytological diagnoses were made on the basis of pro-

nounced cellular and nuclear irregularities, including some mitoses.

Followup of a Lesion by Brushing Cytology

In our laboratory, the brushing method has been employed with biopsy in most cases as a regular followup for various gastroesophageal lesions, regardless of the endoscopic impression, because we occasionally have encountered endoscopically benign-appearing ulcers that proved to be malignant on the histological examination and also to avoid a bias from the endoscopic impression. A malignant ulcer can manifest pronounced healing, almost complete in some cases, only to recur later (195, 197). Such a followup approach, in combination with direct-vision biopsy, is indispensable for detecting a gastroesophageal lesion in its superficial stage when invasion is limited to the mucosa or submucosa.

Simultaneous Biopsy (Table 8.3)

In a series of 50 patients (213), biopsy under direct vision was performed immediately after brushing cytology, in the same endoscopy procedure. In 35 patients

TABLE 8.3

Diagnosis of Gastroesophageal Malignant Tumors
by Combined Use of Biopsy and Cytology
under Direct Vision

Cytology	Biopsy	No. of Cases
Positive	Positive	35
Positive	Negative	10
Negative	Positive	5
Negative	Negative	0

Source: Prolla et al. (213).
Note: N = 50

both biopsy and cytology were positive for malignancy. In 10 patients, cytology was positive and biopsy was negative. In 5 patients, biopsy was positive and cytology was negative. In no patient were both biopsy and cytology negative.

In conclusion, direct-vision cytology of the upper gastrointestinal tract is easily performed during endoscopy and has a high detection rate; combined with biopsy it reduces the sampling error to zero.

Acridine-Orange Fluorescence Microscopy (Table 8.4)

The Acridine-Orange method had a sensitivity of 80%; of the 34 patients with malignant tumors of the upper

TABLE 8.4

ACRIDINE-ORANGE FLUORESCENT MICROSCOPY IN DIRECT-VISION
BRUSHING OF ESOPHAGUS AND STOMACH

Cytology Results	Proved Cancer	Benign Lesions	Total
Positive	27	1	28
"Suspicious"	3	2	5
Negative	3	147	150
Unsatisfactory	1	1	2
Totals	34	151	185

NOTE: N = 185.

gastrointestinal tract seen during the period of the study, 27 had positive Acridine-Orange cytological results. In 5 additional patients, the cells were highly suspicious of malignancy, but could not be designated as positive. In 3 of the cases a malignant tumor was found later. The specificity of the positive report was 96.4%, in close agreement with our specificity rates with the Papanicolaou method.

The detection rate of 80% compares favorably with the published results of other authors (20, 21, 52, 101, 214, 283, 285), using the washing method for collection and Acridine Orange for staining. It is about 10% lower than the direct-vision method stained by Papanicolaou. However, direct comparisons are not valid, because only one or two smears were made for the Acridine-Orange study, whereas six to eight smears are usually made for the routine Papanicolaou staining method.

The detection rate of 80% and the specificity of 96.4% of the positive report, make the method suitable in mass surveys; this potential use is further increased by the ease and rapidity of the staining. The screening also was very rapid, because only one or two smears were made, and they were rich in well-preserved cells. The small number of smears may account for the somewhat lower detection rate, but it should be emphasized that we were interested chiefly in the feasibility of a mass survey tool.

The need for photography as the only source of permanent records of the findings is a disadvantage; only selected groups of cells are recorded, and the procedure increases the cost of the method. The need for special optical equipment for fluorescent microscopy also increases the cost of the method.

In conclusion, the Acridine-Orange method of fluorescent microscopy has reasonably satisfactory accuracy rates, is rapid and easy for cytotechnicians already trained in the more routine methods, and has potential value in mass surveys. Means of decreasing costs should be sought and a reduction in sampling error is desirable.

Shorr's Polychromic Method (Table 8.5)

TABLE 8.5

SHORR'S POLYCHROMIC STAINING IN DIRECT-VISION
BRUSHING OF ESOPHAGUS AND STOMACH

Cytology Results	Proved Cancer	Benign Lesions	Total
Positive	18	0	18
"Suspicious"	3	1	4
Negative	3	97	100
Unsatisfactory	1	1	2
Totals	25	99	124

NOTE: N = 124.

In the search for possible mass survey cytological techniques, a study with the polychromic S3 stain of Shorr also was undertaken.

Of 25 patients with proved malignant tumors of the gastrointestinal tract, 18, or 72%, were positive by the staining method (of direct-vision collection technique). No false-positive result was encountered, giving the positive report a 100% specificity in this relatively small series.

One of the main technical difficulties was to achieve uniformly good nuclear staining. It is our impression that significantly better results were achieved when dimethylsulfoxide (DMSO) was added to the fixative solution (95% ethyl alcohol) to a final concentration of 1%.

Again, only two smears were made for the Shorr technique. One cytopathologist (Dr. Rogerio G. Xavier) made all the readings independently, before any result of the routine cytology was available. As with the Acridine-Orange technique, the aim of the study was to test the feasibility of a potential mass survey tool. The detection rate, as well as the absence of false-positive tests, is encouraging, and a larger study is in progress.

The method appears to have two advantages over Acridine Orange: there is no need for special optical equipment or for photography as a permanent record, which reduces the expense.

9

The Use of Diagnostic Cytology in Mass Surveys for Gastric Carcinoma

In an editorial in *Acta Cytologica,* Dr. George L. Wied (291) of the University of Chicago called attention to the need for careful planning and operation of mass surveys by cytology for the detection of cervical cancer. In certain countries like Japan, Chile, and Germany the incidence and death rates of gastric carcinoma are very high (255), and mass surveys have a definite place. However, to our knowledge only Japan is proceeding with such a program, although cytology is not utilized extensively as a screening method. A thorough review of the techniques for such mass population surveys should be undertaken.

An analysis of the problem indicates that the methods currently in use in Japan have some limitations that may prevent a major expansion of the program. Some of these are as follows:

a) Too many instances of benign conditions are detected for each case of gastric carcinoma. The finding of a high incidence of ulcer or related conditions perhaps should not necessarily represent an achievement, because this is not the prime objective of this program; and the financial resources and time of medical personnel needed to exclude carcinoma in these false-positive cases add considerably to the actual cost of the cancer-finding program.

b) The existing scarcity of physicians limits the use of those methods requiring them, such as endoscopic examinations.

c) The actual and the potential risks of irradiation, especially in unsuspected pregnancy, are a serious drawback of methods utilizing photofluorography.

Exfoliative cytology of the stomach has been considered too time-consuming for practical use in mass surveys for gastric carcinoma. But this may not necessarily be correct.

The first point is that in any such method, complete and elaborate planning is needed. A program already exists for cervical cancer screening; it can easily be adapted to other areas like gastric carcinoma. In 1961, the United States Health Service created the so-called Fourteen-Step Project for Cervical Cancer Screening Projects. This very important work can be adapted to similar programs, as in gastric carcinoma screening. These fourteen steps are listed specifically as follows, and discussion of them is taken from Wied's editorial (291):

1. Planning
2. Orientation of essential project personnel
3. Enlistment of patients
4. Orientation of patients
5. Initial collection of patient information
6. Collection of the cytologic material
7. Cytological examinations
8. Followup of significant cytology
9. Complete workup of significant cytology cases
10. Tissue diagnosis
11. Clinical diagnosis
12. Treatment
13. Periodic followup of patients with negative cytology
14. Evaluation of the program

All cancers must be proved by tissue examination and eventually treated in such a manner that the lesion is eradicated. Failure in any of these steps would largely negate the advantage of good-quality cytology and the accomplishment of early detection. The patient then must be followed for a reasonable period of time for evidence of persistent or recurrent cancer.

In Japan, for example, the time seems appropriate for a unification of efforts of cytologists and clinicians at a cancer center in a large city to initiate a pilot program along the lines of the fourteen-step project. "Step 1—Planning" is one of the most important, and careful study should be undertaken before any action is done. Without this planning, the entire program is in jeopardy and may fail completely, with enormous losses in financial resources and time of medical and paramedical personnel, not to mention unrealized hopes for the control of gastric carcinoma.

We should now consider in some detail four of the questions raised in step 1.

1. *What is known about the population in terms of incidence and death rates from carcinoma of the stomach within the past several years?*

Japan already has a considerable amount of information on death rates from gastric carcinoma, accumulated by the efforts of Professor Segi and his collaborators at Tohoku University (255). These data indicate that Japan has a very high death rate from gastric carcinoma, without indications of any decline. For the entire male population (all ages), in the period 1962–63, the rate was 57.32 per 100,000. However, the tables of Professor Segi reveal a sharp increase in the rates starting at 40 to 50 years of age, for both males and females, as follows (1962–63 data):

Males, age 40–44 . . . . . . 31.83 per 100,000
Males, age 45–49 . . . . . . 62.95 per 100,000
Males, age 50–54 . . . . .113.76 per 100,000
Males, age 55–59 . . . . .194.34 per 100,000
Males, age 60–64 . . . . . .308.11 per 100,000
. . . .
Males, age 75–79 . . . . . .609.28 per 100,000 (peak rate)

Females, age 40–44 . . . . 28.80 per 100,000
Females, age 45–49 . . . . 42.73 per 100,000
Females, age 50–54 . . . . 65.63 per 100,000
Females, age 55–59 . . . . 94.03 per 100,000
. . . .
Females, age 75–79 . . . .323.06 per 100,000 (peak rate)

This pattern is in curious contrast to other countries, such as the United States, where gastric carcinoma is in decline, for reasons not known at present. It is possible that this trend has something to do with improvement in the general health of the population. In the United States, this steady decrease (in both sexes) of the age-adjusted rate of death from gastric carcinoma makes any attempt at mass surveys highly impractical and costly.

2. *What has been undertaken in the past on control of carcinoma of the stomach, and how efficient were these programs?*

Japan already has initiated mass surveys for the control of gastric carcinoma, and Ariga (6) has reviewed the experience of his country on this subject. However, exfoliative cytology has not been used in such programs. The main methods in 51 programs were:
   a) Photofluorography, with or without clinical interview, 42 programs
   b) Photofluorography plus gastrocamera and interview, 4 programs
Such programs examined 333,531 persons in 1965, and 455,078 persons in 1966. This is a positive, although modest, beginning when one considers that according to the 1965 census in Japan there were 29,068,514 persons over forty years of age.

It is difficult to evaluate the efficiency of these pro-

grams from the available literature and information. A point in favor of such programs is the impressive number of gastric carcinomas, many at the early stage, disclosed by such screening. In 1965, 538 cases were found, and in 1966, 432 cases. However, this result was achieved at the high price of a detailed examination of 33,902 persons (10.2% of the entire population screened) in 1965, and 39.791 persons (8.7%) in 1966. This effort seems excessive, and maintaining such percentages would require the detailed examination of about three million persons over forty years of age to complement the screening of such a population. This excessive rate of false-positives of almost 80 noncancer cases for each cancer case adds enormously to the cost of the cancer-finding program.

The other parameter of efficiency, the accuracy rate, is not apparent from the available data. Information is lacking on the followup of a significant sample of the negative cases. Another approach is to calculate, however grossly, the detection rate—that is, to plot the expected number of gastric carcinomas in the screened population against the actual number of cases found. In the data of the 1965 and 1966 surveys, if one assumes that all people examined (788,609) were forty years of age or over, and distributed in age and sex as in the respective general populations, the expected number of cases would be approximately 1,200. The actual number was 970, that is, 80%. This, however, is an assumption, because we do not know the age and sex distribution of the population screened. If, by another example, the populations were over forty-five years of age, the expected number would be 1,450 and the 970 cases found would represent now only 67%. Such an analysis seems desirable for an objective assessment of the methods in use. However, as we will note later, there are reasons other than efficiency which limit such methods.

3. *Are the incidence and mortality rates high enough to justify such mass surveys? Will the yield be high enough to keep the cost per case reasonably low?*

An ideal population group to screen for gastric carcinoma should yield at least a 2 per 1,000 detection rate and account for at least 90% of all gastric carcinomas occurring in the entire population.

The incidence of 45.90 per 100,000 of the entire population of Japan is not sufficiently high to allow such a detection rate; the mass screening of the entire population would give a detection rate of only 1 per 2,000.

As was noted earlier, the tables published by Segi and Kwishara (255) show a sharp increase in the death rates starting at forty years of age. This can be used as the first means of increasing the detection rate. Using the 1965 official census of the Japanese population and the rates established by Segi and Kurihara for the period 1962–63, it is apparent that the Japanese population over forty years of age comprises 29,068,514 persons (29.57% of the entire population), and that it accounts for 97.84% of all gastric carcinoma deaths, having a rate of 152.19 per 100,000. The screening of such population at random would give a maximum detection rate of 1.5 cases per 1,000 persons screened, still short of an ideal group.

Similar calculations for the Japanese population of forty-five years of age or over reveal 23,107,112 persons (23.51% of the total population), and indicate that this group accounts for 93.9% of all gastric carcinoma deaths, having a rate of 183.65 per 100,000. The screening of such a population would give a maximum detection rate of 1.8 cases per 1,000 persons screened, very close to the theoretically ideal situation. Calculations made for the Japanese population of fifty years of age or over totaled 18,185,301 persons (18.54% of the total population), and indicated that this group accounts for 88.21% of all gastric carcinomas, having a rate of 219.37 per 100,000. The screening at random would give a maximum detection rate of 2.1 cases per 1,000 persons screened. This group has a detection rate above the ideal, but accounts for less (however slightly) than 90% of the gastric carcinomas. Attempting to increase the detection rate by simply augmenting the age at which screening starts, from this point on, would have two serious disadvantages: first, the percentage of gastric carcinomas encompassed by the screening would be significantly less than 90%, and the highly productive —with reasonable life expectancy—group of people between forty and forty-five and over fifty-five would not benefit from the screening.

In conclusion, the ideal screening group cannot be found by age-group criteria only. The age group of forty-five years and over, however, appears to be a reasonable compromise. Another important question that remains is the ideal time interval between reexamina-tions of the same persons within a specific age group.

4. *What is the best screening method for mass surveys?*

This is a very difficult question. Theoretically, there are three main procedures for such mass surveys: (*a*) photofluorography; (*b*) gastrocamera; and (*c*) cytology.

The use of photofluorography (the method most widely employed in Japan at present) has serious drawbacks that eventually will prevent a major expansion of such programs there. They already have caused such surveys to be abandoned in the United States. The main objections to such methods are the high number of false-positive cases, the need for physicians, and the problem of radiation. For each case of gastric carcinoma detected in Japan, there were almost 80 instances of benign conditions. The cost of studying such cases in detail soon will be a significant deterrent to the cancer-finding program. And even if the cost could be reduced in one way or another, the hospital facilities of the involved communities would be almost paralyzed by such efforts. A hospital serving a community of 250,000 persons, screening all people forty-five years of age or older, would have to admit approximately 5,000 patients for detailed examinations to detect little more than sixty cases of gastric carcinoma.

A second problem of photofluorography of the stomach is that it requires the presence of physicians. However, this problem may be more or less easily solved because radiology technicians probably can be trained to do the examination entirely without the assistance of a radiologist.

A third criticism is the problem of radiation effects in large segments of the population. First of all, it should be remembered that damage from radiation tends to be cumulative, especially in relationship to *genetic* effects, and that no true dose threshold (a dose below which there is no effect) can be found. The genetic effect upon future generations is relevant to the mass survey problem, where a relatively large dose of radiation is delivered to a large segment of the population. All these considerations should be seriously examined by the Japanese medical profession before a major expansion of the already extensive use of photofluorography of the stomach is accepted as appropriate medical practice. If such surveys are to be continued, the Japanese population should receive all possible protection, especially in mandatory gonadal shielding for people in the reproductive age and in avoiding exposure of pregnant women to radiation. The ten-day interval following the onset of menstruation is the only time when it is virtually certain that women of such age are not pregnant. During the period from two to six weeks of pregnancy, the embryo is especially sensitive to radiation.

Several mass surveys for gastric carcinoma, using photofluorography, have been undertaken in the United States. They were all abandoned, mainly because of the radiation hazard and the decreasing death rate of gastric carcinoma in the United States. It is interesting that the results were comparable to those reported more recently by the Japanese investigators. In the study of Roach, Sloan, and Morgan (231), 10,000 cases were studied by photofluorography of the stomach; in 9,072 instances a satisfactory study was achieved, of which 9.4%, or 853 cases, were read as abnormal, requiring detailed examination, and 27 cases of proved gastric malignancy were found (a detection rate of 2.7 per 1,000). In this study, six photofluorographs were taken from each patient in recumbent position, and no fluoroscopy was used. It was calculated that 0.5 to 2.0 R were delivered to the patient's skin at each film.

In the study of Wigh and Swenson (294), 5,340 cases were examined by photofluorography, 81.4% with a 70-mm Schmidt-Helm camera. Six exposures were made of each patient, with a total dosage of 4 to 12 R at the skin. A total of 7,075 examinations were done on these 5,430 persons, of which 6,566 (92.8%) were considered satisfactory; 322 (4.9%) were read as abnormal, and regular gastrointestinal X-ray examination was recommended. Twelve cases of gastric neoplasms were found, of which 3 were proved gastric carcinomas (a detection rate of only 0.6 per 1,000).

In summary, photofluorography appears to be a less than satisfactory method for mass surveys for gastric carcinoma; the false-positive cases are too frequent and the hazard of radiation, especially genetic, appears to be significant.

Two methods remain: exfoliative cytology and gastrocamera endoscopy. A carefully planned study should be undertaken by a university or cancer center in Japan to compare the two methods and to determine their roles in the mass survey for gastric carcinoma. A significant study should probably include 10,000 cases, preferably people forty-five years of age or over, studied by each method, with a detailed analysis of the results of each series, giving respective detection rates, true-positive/false-positive ratios, cost per case of carcinoma, and personnel and equipment needs, and answering other pertinent questions. As Wied (292) has indicated, computers would be of great help in a study of this magnitude because of the enormous needs for data storage and retrieval. Only after such prospective study can proper emphasis be placed upon one or the other method, or any combination of such methods.

10
Duodenal Drainage (Secretin Test) and Cytology

Carcinomas of the pancreas and biliary tree are usually very difficult to diagnose with certainty before exploratory laparotomy, and the prognosis remains very poor. The great majority of patients die within a year after the diagnosis.

The pancreas is not accessible to direct investigation, and usually is evaluated by changes in the neighboring organs. Only very recently have more direct approaches to the pancreas been designed. Pancreatic scannings by radioisotopes are still of very little use owing to the high rate of nonspecific findings. Pancreatography is still in its infancy, but Japanese reports of endoscopic pancreatography by cannulation of the papilla major are of considerable interest. The recent development of safe and practical fiberoptic duodenoscopes opens new possibilities for direct-vision cytology and biopsy.

The technique of duodenal intubation for biliary and pancreatic secretion studies deserves wider use because the cytological examination of the secretion obtained is rewarding in about 60% of patients with cancer of the pancreas. This percentage is relatively small when compared with other areas of the digestive tract, but this contribution to the evaluation of a difficult problem is still useful. The present chapter reviews our total experience with duodenal drainage, including the previously published data of Raskin et al. (221, 224), to delineate its clinical importance in the diagnosis of carcinoma of the biliary tree and pancreas, as well as in the diagnosis of chronic pancreatitis.

Material

During the period between April 1955 and December 1968, 2,521 duodenal drainages were performed; in 25, the material was collected only for microbiological studies, leaving a total of 2,496 drainages for cytologic studies. These 2,496 procedures were accomplished in 2,181 patients, all of whom were followed for a minimum of twelve months. The group of 2,181 patients is composed of 182 with proved malignant tumors of the biliary tract, pancreas, and duodenum, and 1,999 with proved benign lesions or negative followup, all adults. As with other areas of the digestive tract, the data include only the initial examination, except when the first study proved unsatisfactory and a repeat examination was made within two weeks.

Cytology Results

Accuracy

The results are condensed in table 10.1. Of the 182 malignant tumors, 107 were correctly diagnosed, a sensitivity of 58.7%. In 9 patients, or 5% of the total number of cases of malignant tumors, the drainage tube could not be advanced beyond the duodenal bulb or the first few centimeters of the descending duodenum.

TABLE 10.1
DIAGNOSTIC ACCURACY OF DUODENAL DRAINAGE CYTOLOGY

Lesion	Patients	Positive Cytology	Positive Report Analysis	Negative Cytology	Unsatisfactory [a]
Clinically benign lesion or normal hepatopancreatic area	1,999	5 [b]	*Specificity* 95.6%	1,950	39
Proved malignant lesions			*Sensitivity*		
Pancreas	156	90	—	66	—
Hepatobiliary tree	18	9		9	—
Duodenum	8	8	—	—	—
Total	182	107	58.7%	75	—

NOTE: University of Chicago, April 1955 to 30 December 1968; 2,181 patients.
[a] Not repeated.
[b] In 5 additional patients a malignant tumor was found in another area (see text).

In 5 such cases, the duodenal wash at the point where the tube resisted advance was positive for malignant cells. In the other patients, the wash was negative for malignant cells; these cases have been arbitrarily classified as false-negatives, but they could well be classified as unsatisfactory tests. Using this criterion, no unsatisfactory examination was encountered in the group of malignant tumors (and actually only one case had a positive report after an initial unsatisfactory test done a few days before).

The 1,999 patients free of cancer in the biliary tract, duodenum and pancreas were correctly diagnosed as negative in 1,950 instances, whereas 39 had unsatisfactory tests not repeated and 10 had positive cytology. In 5 of the false-positive tests, a malignant tumor was found in another area (3 gastric carcinomas, 1 esophageal tumor, and 1 lung carcinoma), and the false-positive test thus helped to focus attention upon the presence of a neoplasm. In the other 5 cases, no tumor was found anywhere, and the false-positive test was clinically misleading.

The 10 false-positive cytology reports represent 0.5% of the total number of patients with negative followup, and the 5 instances of false-positive with totally negative followup represents 4.4% of the positive reports. The specificity of the positive report, therefore, is of the order of 95.6%.

Correlation between the Cytologic and Histopathologic Findings

All 182 malignant tumors were adenocarcinomas. Isolated signet-ring cells were seen on only one occasion, the cytologic presentation usually consisting of clumps or clusters of adenocarcinoma type cells. In 2 patients, some cells closely resembled squamous-cell carcinoma type, and indeed the histology showed pronounced squamous metaplasia of the tumor. In 2 additional instances, the cells were of the squamous type and a tumor elsewhere was mentioned as the first possibility; tumors were found in the esophagus and in the lung.

Location of the Tumor and the Cytology Result

As is seen in table 10.1, the vast majority of the tumors were located in the pancreas (156 patients), while 18 were located in the biliary tree and 8 in the duodenum (6 primary tumors and 2 metastatic lesions). Of the pancreatic tumors, 90, or about 60%, were in the head and body of the pancreas; 44, or approximately 30%, were in the body or body and tail of the pancreas, 12 were in the tail of the pancreas, and 10 were too advanced for proper classification and involved the entire gland and adjacent organs.

Analysis of the series in such groups, already arbitrary, nevertheless reflects little of the accuracy in the various subgroups because of the wide variation in size of these subgroups. If anything, carcinomas of the head of the pancreas and carcinomas of the duodenum appear to be the most easily diagnosed by cytology, whereas tumors of the biliary tree, body, and tail of the pancreas, in that order, are much more difficult to recognize, as would be anticipated.

Volume and Bicarbonate Concentration after Secretin Stimulation

From April 1955 to December 1968, our laboratory had considerable experience with secretin-stimulated duodenal drainage. However, because several different lots and brands of secretin were employed, the entire series is not homogeneous and comparisons or correlations between tests done in 1955 and 1968, for example, are not necessarily valid. Because Dr. Howard F. Raskin published his experience up to 1959 (221, 224) and because during 1960–61 we used a preparation from Eli Lilly Laboratory which is no longer available, in the following discussion we consider only the results for the period 1962 to 1968. Also, since 1962 we have mainly employed the preparation of Jorpes from Sweden; this preparation has been remarkably constant in potency.

The results are condensed in tables 10.2, 10.3, and

TABLE 10.2
DUODENAL DRAINAGE: SECRETIN TEST

Total Volumes (ml/kg/30′)	No. of Cases	Percentage	Cumulative Percentage
0.49 or less	28	2.32	2.32
0.50 to 0.89	106	8.79	11.11
0.90 to 1.29	336	27.86	38.97
1.30 to 1.69	388	32.17	71.14
1.70 to 2.09	190	15.75	86.89
2.10 to 2.49	86	7.13	94.02
2.50 to 2.89	39	3.22	97.24
2.90 to 3.29	16	1.32	98.56
3.30 to 3.69	9	0.75	99.31
3.70 to 4.09	4	0.33	99.64
4.10 or more	4	0.33	99.97
Total	1,206	—	100.00

NOTE: Mean: 1.44; S.D.: 0.54; Mean ± 2 S.D.: 0.36 to 2.52.

10.4. In table 10.2 the results are tabulated for the 1,206 procedures performed during the above-mentioned period, for the total volume, expressed in ml/kg/30′, as well as the percentages (individual and cumulative values). The mean total volume was 1.44 ml/kg/30′, with a standard deviation of 0.54. The mean plus or minus two standard deviations gives a range of 0.36 to 2.52 ml/kg/30′. In table 10.2, Hoffmann's method (116) for plotting the results was used. The normal values range between 0.50 and 1.69 ml/kg/30′. However, a random distribution also was noted in the values between 2.50 and 4.09 ml/kg/30′. Patients with liver disease (cirrhosis, viral hepatitis, fatty change, hemosiderosis, and hemochromatosis) accounted for such distribution. The normal values for patients with liver disease are in that high range. A similar analysis was attempted with volume values less than 0.50, but

Material and Results at the
University of Chicago

TABLE 10.3

Duodenal Drainage: Secretin Test

(*Distribution of HCO₃—Maximal Values [mEq/L]*)

mEq/L	No. of Cases	Percent	Cumulative Percent
Less than 30	23	2.0	2.0
30–39	24	2.0	4.0
40–49	36	3.0	7.0
50–59	34	2.8	9.8
60–69	50	4.1	13.9
70–79	101	8.3	22.2
80–89	133	11.0	33.2
90–99	415	34.5	67.7
100–109	282	23.3	91.0
110–19	92	7.6	98.6
120 or over	16	1.3	99.9
Total	1,206	—	100.0

Note: Mean: 88 mEq/L; S.D.: 8.5 mEq/L; Mean ± 2 S.D.: 71 to 105 mEq/L.

no normal distribution was detected. It is interesting that, of the 28 cases with a volume of 0.45 ml/kg/30' or less (table 10.4), 15 were instances of carcinoma of the pancreas, 4 were chronic pancreatitis, and 9 comprised a miscellaneous range of diagnoses, but probably had a normal pancreas (probably representing errors inherent in the technique itself). The discrimination between carcinoma and pancreatitis cannot be made on the basis of the total volume of duodenal aspirate alone.

In table 10.3 we have tabulated the values of bi-carbonate concentration, expressed in mEq per liter, in the same 1,206 procedures. The mean bicarbonate concentration of the peak value was 88 mEq/L, with a standard deviation of 8.5. The mean plus or minus two standard deviations gives a range of 71 to 105 mEq/L. In table 10.3, Hoffmann's method for plotting the results was used. Again, two ranges of random distribution were noted. The normal values are represented by the figures exceeding 71 mEq/L, and a second random distribution was noted for the values less than 50 mEq/L. Of the 83 patients with bicarbonate concentrations of 49 mEq/L or less (table 10.4), 23 had carcinoma of the pancreas, 5 had chronic pancreatitis histologically proved or strongly suggested by the clinical history and radiological findings; the remaining 55 cases had a miscellaneous range of diseases and probably normal pancreatic function (technical error?). Again, a low bicarbonate concentration cannot discriminate between carcinoma of the pancreas and chronic pancreatitis; and a value of low bicarbonate (here defined as 49 mEq/L or less) was observed in more instances of cancer than of pancreatitis.

Sensitivity and Specificity of Total Volume, Bicarbonate Concentration, and the Combination of the Two Values

The initial hope when the secretin test was designed was that it would delineate normal and abnormal pancreatic secretion rates, with additional discrimination of

TABLE 10.4

Specificity and Sensitivity of the Low Values in the Secretin Test

Diagnosis	Patients	HCO₃ below 50 mEq/L (83 Patients)		Total Volume below 0.49 ml/kg/30' (28 Patients)		Both Values Low (16 Patients)	
		No. of Patients	Specificity [a] Sensitivity [b]	No. of Patients	Specificity Sensitivity	No. of Patients	Specificity Sensitivity
Chronic pancreatitis	14	5	SP: 5/83 or 6% SEN: 5/14 or 35%	4	SP: 4/28 or 14% SEN: 4/14 or 28%	2	SP: 2/16 or 12.5% SEN: 2/14 or 14%
Carcinoma of pancreas and biliary tree	50	23	SP: 23/83 or 27% SEN: 23/50 or 46%	15	SP: 15/28 or 53% SEN: 15/50 or 30%	12 [c]	SP: 12/16 or 75% SEN: 12/50 or 24%
"Controls"	1,142	55	Nonspecific percentage: 66%	9	Nonspecific percentage: 33%	2	Nonspecific percentage: 12.5%
Total	1,206	83	—	28	—	16	—

Note: University of Chicago, January 1962 to 31 December 1968; 1,206 patients.
[a] Specificity is defined as the percentage of the abnormal values that are caused by the respective pathological processes.
[b] Sensitivity is defined as the percentage of cases with the respective pathological processes that have abnormal value.
[c] All 12 cases were carcinomas of the pancreas.

the abnormal results caused by carcinoma from those resulting from pancreatitis. Cancer of the pancreas was presumed to be indicated by reduced volumes (of less than 1.1 ml/kg/30′) with normal or low bicarbonate concentration (then defined as less than 90 mEq/L). Chronic pancreatitis was characterized by normal volumes and low bicarbonate concentrations. The present series does not confirm any of the above correlations because the specificity of such values is extremely low (table 10.4).

Total Volumes of 1.1 ml/kg/30′

Our data show clearly that the low limit of the normal total volume is 0.50 ml/kg/30′ and not 1.1 as previously indicated. Analysis of the cases with total volumes of 1.1 ml/kg/30′ or less revealed that only 15% of such cases had pancreaticobiliary carcinomas (too low a degree of specificity to be of any value).

Bicarbonate Concentration Less Than 90 mEq/L

Our data indicate that the low limit of the normal bicarbonate concentration is 71 mEq/L and not 90, as previously indicated. Moreover, an analysis of the patients with bicarbonate concentrations less than 90 mEq/L revealed 12% of such cases with pancreaticobiliary carcinomas and 3% with chronic pancreatitis proved histologically or strongly suggested by the clinical findings and radiology; again, the specificity is too low and also fails to discriminate between cancer and pancreatitis.

Total Volume Less Than 1.1 ml/kg/30′ and Bicarbonate Concentration Less Than 90 mEq/L

This combination of the two parameters was slightly more definitive for carcinoma than either alone; 19% of such cases had pancreaticobiliary carcinomas, still too low a figure to be of diagnostic value.

Total Volume of 0.49 ml/kg/30′ or Less

Having established the low limit of the total volume as 0.50 ml/kg/30′, we studied those patients with volumes below such levels. As was indicated previously, 15 of 28 such cases had carcinoma of the pancreas, a specificity of 53%. This percentage is better than the 15% of the 1.1 ml/kg/30′ volumes, but still too low to be of significant diagnostic value. Also, 4 patients, or approximately 14%, had pancreatitis; in summary, 67%

of such values are distinctly abnormal, and the changes are more evident for cancer than for pancreatitis.

Bicarbonate Concentration of 49 mEq/L or Less

As was indicated previously, 23 of 83 such cases, or 27%, had carcinoma and 5, or only 6%, had proved or highly probable chronic pancreatitis. In summary, 33% of such values are definitively abnormal (carcinoma or pancreatitis) but the discrimination was inadequate.

Total Volume Less Than 0.50 ml/kg/30′ with Bicarbonate Concentration Less Than 50 mEq/L

In 16 patients, both the volume and the bicarbonate concentration were below the minimum for clinical normal values. In 12, or about 80%, of such cases the diagnosis was carcinoma of the pancreas; in 2 patients, chronic calcific pancreatitis; and in 2 instances the pancreas was probably normal and heavy contamination with bile was noted during the test (both patients had cirrhosis of the liver).

Conclusions

From these data and from the statistical analysis summarized in tables 10.2, 10.3, and 10.4, the following practical conclusions seem warranted:

a) The lower limits of bicarbonate concentration for adults are 71 mEq/L (mean minus two standard deviations). However, even values *below 50 mEq/L* have too low a degree of sensitivity to be of clinical value.

b) The normal range for adults of total volume (mean plus or minus two standard deviations) is 0.36 to 2.52 ml/kg/30′, whereas the gaussian curve of clinical tests gives a range of 0.50 to 1.69 ml/kg/30′.

c) Total volumes below 0.50 ml/kg/30′ accounted for carcinoma of the pancreas in 53% of cases and chronic pancreatitis in 14%.

d) Values of 2.50 ml/kg/30′ or more of total volumes are due in 80% of the instances to hepatic disease (especially cirrhosis, fatty degeneration, and hepatitis).

e) Exfoliative cytology is positive in 58.7% of carcinomas of the duodenum, pancreas, and biliary tree.

f) Such carcinomas have a total volume of 0.49 ml/kg/30′ or less in 30% of the instances, and a bicarbonate concentration of 49 mEq/L or less in 46%.

g) Approximately 80% of the patients with a total volume of 49 ml/kg/30′ or less *and* bicarbonate con-

**Material and Results at the
University of Chicago**

centration of 49 mEq/L or less have carcinoma of the pancreas.

Comments and Review of the Literature

Cytology Results

Cytological examination of duodenal aspirates (after sample aspiration or washings, or stimulation with secretin or magnesium sulfate) has not been used widely (table 10.5). However occasional case reports, published in the late 1940s, attest to the possibility of identifying malignant cells in the duodenal contents (173, 174).

TABLE 10.5

CYTOLOGY RESULTS IN DUODENAL DRAINAGE AND SECRETIN TEST

Authors	No. of Patients with Cancer	Positive Cytology	Detection Rate	Specificity of Positive Cytology
Bowden and Papanicolaou (33)	46	22	47%	95.7%
Dreiling, Nieburgs, and Janowitz (67)	60	47	78%	75.0%
Ishioka (122)	81	47	42%	Not stated
Goldstein and Ventzke (95)	24	18	75%	100.0%
University of Chicago				
Raskin et al. (221)	55	33	60%	94.3%
Present series [a]	182	107	58%	95.6%

NOTE: *Series selected from the literature.*
[a] Includes Raskin's cases.

Lemon and Byrnes (41,159–61) were the first to report a reasonably large series, using mainly aspiration of the duodenal contents, and occasionally stimulation with secretin or a 33.3% solution of magnesium sulfate. In 1951, Lemon (159) reported positive cytology in two-thirds of 55 patients with proved carcinoma of the pancreas or biliary tract. He also noted 3% false-positive diagnoses in 85 patients without cancer, and a 7% incidence of unsatisfactory tests. In a previous paper (160), the same authors reported 27% "questionable" smears, making analysis of the entire series very difficult, if not impossible. In 1954 (41), Byrnes and Lemon reported a series of 151 tests; malignant cells were identified in 13 of 36 patients with proved carcinoma, a detection rate of 36%.

The group working with Papanicolaou first reported their experience in 1951 (257): in 68 patients having duodenal or biliary tract drainage studies, 21 had proved

carcinomas, 10 were diagnosed or suspected by smear, and there was 1 false-positive. In 1960, Bowden and Papanicolaou (33) reported 22 positive diagnoses, representing 47% of 46 cases of proved carcinomas. As in most of Papanicolaou's work, the use of class III complicates analysis of the data for clinical significance. In 1959 (32), the same authors reported on the cellular study of aspiration of the pancreatic duct of Wirsung during the Whipple operation. Malignant cells were recognized in 7 of 12 cases with pancreatic carcinoma. This is an interesting approach and should be compared with pancreatic biopsy in a controlled prospective study.

A similar approach has been reported by Rosen, Garrett, and Aka (232). In 21 patients suspected of pancreatic carcinoma, 16 subsequently had proved malignancy. In 5 cases, malignant cells were collected by trans-operational ductal aspiration, and in 6 additional patients a class III ("suspicious") report was issued.

The group at the Mount Sinai Hospital in New York has accumulated considerable experience with duodenal drainage after secretin stimulation (63–67, 188). Their cytologic results were first published in 1960 (67): 47 positive tests of 60 patients with carcinoma of the pancreas and positive tests in each of 7 patients with biliary tract carcinoma. However, they reported an unusually high incidence of false-positive diagnoses: 12 instances. This finding and the emphasis upon the so-called malignant associated changes complicate the clinical significance of their results. In 1962 (188), "malignant associated changes" (MAC) were noted in the cells of 68 patients after duodenal drainage: 48 indeed had carcinomas (29 pancreatic and 19 elsewhere), whereas 20 did not have any tumor.

In Europe, Henning and Witte (108, 110–12) have published extensively on the use of cytological examination of the duodenal drainage material. However, no statistical analysis of their cytological material is available for adequate comparison and comment.

In Japan, Ishioka (122) has the widest experience with cytology of duodenal drainage. He reported a detection rate of 42% in a series of 81 patients with proved carcinoma. No mention was made of false-positive or benign cases. He also developed a technique of direct aspiration of the gallbladder or biliary ducts during laparoscopy. In a series of 42 malignant tumors, 13 were cytologically positive. Of the 8 carcinomas of the gallbladder, 7 were positive—a remarkable result.

Another interesting approach was devised by Klavins and Flemma (137) in 1964, by the cytological study of bile aspirated during percutaneous transhepatic cholangiography.

The first report by the group at the University of Chicago was a case report in 1953 on the cytologic diagnosis of a malignant lymphoma (histiocytic type) of the duodenum, by Goldgraber, Rubin, and Owens (94). They also described their method of intubation, using a slight modification of Lemon's technique. In the same year, Rubin et al. (243) published a small series using this method. Duodenal cytology was correctly negative in 27 proved benign cases. The series included two malignancies each of the liver, bile ducts, and gallbladder, all missed by cytology. However, 4 of 8 carcinomas of the pancreas were diagnosed by cytology.

In April 1955, Raskin initiated the technique used since then in our laboratory (described in detail in chap. 3). There were significant advances in the use of the double-lumen diamond tube and the availability of secretin and cholecystokinin as stimulants for pancreatic and bile flow, respectively. The first report on this technique was published in 1958 (224) and included the results of 203 such duodenal intubations. Carcinoma was demonstrated later in 43 patients, and cytology was positive in 28 instances, a detection rate of 65%. Again, it should be emphasized that cytologic material always was interpreted as either positive or negative for malignancy, without "suspicious" or other intermediary classifications.

The all-inclusive series of 182 malignant tumors reported here has a detection rate of 58.7% (107 positive cytological examinations), not significantly different from the earlier report. The incidence of false-positive reports is similarly low; only 5 truly false-positive instances (in 5 additional cases a malignant tumor was found elsewhere, explaining the presence of the malignant cells).

The detection rate of 58.7% is a worthwhile accomplishment in an area presenting as much diagnostic difficulty as the pancreaticobiliary tract. However, further diagnostic improvements should be sought to permit earlier diagnosis. A continuation of immunological screening followed by duodenal drainage cytology (complemented, we hope, by direct-vision procedures by means of the duodenoscope) should bring us closer to this goal.

Secretin Test

Study of the total volume of pancreatic secretion and its bicarbonate concentration after stimulation with secretin can be a useful complement to the cytological examination if its limitations are properly recognized. Determinations of protein content or enzymatic activity or both are less reliable as parameters of pancreatic exocrine functional status, with the exception of cystic fibrosis (86). It is always difficult to prevent contamination by gastric and intestinal juices, and validation of the recovery rate by markers was not accomplished until recently (89).

Several other points are worth discussing in relation to the secretin test: secretin dose, duration of the test, normal values of total volume, and bicarbonate secretin.

Secretin Dose. Pure natural secretin, available from Jorpes (GIH Research Unit, Chemistry Department, Karolinska Institute, Stockholm, Sweden) has a remarkably constant potency (205). The recommended dose is 1 clinical unit per kg of body weight, injected intravenously during a period of about 3 to 5 min. The studies of Petersen (205), with pure natural secretin from the GIH Research Unit of the Karolinska Institute, showed that the dose of 1 clinical unit per kg of body weight, given in a single intravenous injection, elicits a *nearly maximal* response that lasts for at least 2 hr. During the first hour, the outputs of bicarbonate are nearly constant. In the second postsecretin hour the bicarbonate outputs are, on an average, 61% of those in the first hour.

Duration of Test. Our laboratory performs a 30-min test, with collections fractioned into three samples of 10 min duration each. Dreiling (63–67) uses an 80-min collection period, whereas Bockus, Lopusniak, and Tachdjian (27) prefer a 60-min collection.

The peak secretory response occurs in about 10 to 15 min, and the best clinical correlation is with peak concentration of bicarbonate rather than with absolute amounts. The volume of the pancreatic secretion flow is related to the body weight (205) and should be so correlated. It is our impression, from the literature, that the total volume after 60 or 80 min has the same clinical significance, and in our own experience very little appears to be gained diagnostically from prolonging the test beyond 30 min.

Material and Results at the
University of Chicago

The fractionation into 10-min samples is important to minimize the effects of intermittent contamination with gastric juice or bile upon the bicarbonate concentration. To further minimize contamination with bile, we have recently been stimulating the gallbladder to empty with a dose of cholecystokinin before the secretin test.

Normal Values of Total Volume and Bicarbonate Concentration. In the first report by this laboratory (290), a total volume of at least 1.1 ml/kg/30′ and a bicarbonate concentration of at least 90 mEq/L in one of any of the three collection samples were established as the lower limits of normal pancreatic exocrine secretion under secretin stimulation (1 unit per kg of body weight dose).

This interpretation was based on the study of 108 patients in whom pancreatic disease was thought to be absent, and in whom there was a mean volume of 2.0 ml per kg per 30 min with a standard deviation of 0.9 ml. It is obvious that the mean minus *one* standard deviation is too small a range for establishing the lower limit of the value of a clinical test. As was seen above, only 15% of the patients with less than 1.1 ml per kg per 30 min have carcinoma. On the other hand, the relatively large standard deviation in the series (0.9 ml) made it almost useless to consider 0.2 ml as the lower limit; only an insignificant number of cases would have such values, and the clinical usefulness of the test is diminished greatly. The value 1.1 ml was obviously a compromise—unfortunately, not an accurate one.

The bicarbonate concentration of 90 mEq/L was based on the study of 137 patients with probable absence of pancreatic disease. This group had a mean value of 109 mEq/L, with a standard deviation of 13 mEq. Inasmuch as the bicarbonate concentration appeared to be in close agreement with previous studies (61, 64, 65, 154, 157), the conclusion was reached that 90 mEq/L represented the lower limits of stimulated pancreatic flow. However, the frequent contamination by bile was not seriously considered, and our studies in a much larger number of cases demonstrate that only values below 50 mEq/L have clinical significance, if any.

Clinical Interpretation of the Test. A low volume (less than 1.1 ml/kg/30′) was considered by Raskin et al. (290) the most reliable index to pancreatic duct obstruction resulting from tumor. This was observed in 20 of the 32 cases of pancreatic carcinoma. However, the low specificity of such volume values significantly decreases the clinical value of the test. A concomitant reduction of bicarbonate concentration (values below 90 mEq/L) also occurred in 20 patients with cancer. Again, the low specificity of such a combined set of parameters was not realized (only 19% of such combination of "low" values have pancreaticobiliary carcinoma).

A normal volume with reduced bicarbonate concentration has been considered more characteristic of chronic pancreatitis, according to Dornberger (62) and Dreiling and his group (63–67). However, in all series the number of cases with proved chronic pancreatitis has been small. In our experience, in 14 cases with proved chronic pancreatitis (either by biopsy or the demonstration of calcifications in the area of the pancreas associated with a confirmatory clinical history), only 4 cases had volumes of 0.49 ml/kg/30′ or less, and 5 had bicarbonate concentrations of 49 mEq/L or less. Of these, two had both low volume and bicarbonate concentrations. It is interesting that the bicarbonate concentration was below two standard deviations of the mean (71 mEq/L or less) in 11 of 14 such cases, or 80%. Reduced bicarbonate concentration, therefore, is the most common abnormality in chronic pancreatitis. Unfortunately, only very few cases are below the lower "clinical" normal values, and thus no discrimination between pancreatitis and carcinoma is possible.

High volumes (with normal bicarbonate concentration) above two standard deviations of the mean (2.52 ml/kg/30′) were observed in 63 patients. In 50 patients (or approximately 80%), histological proof of liver disease was obtained: cirrhosis, fatty degeneration, or hepatitis. In 7 patients, diseases frequently associated with liver abnormalities were present (nontropical sprue with severe malnutrition in 4, chronic ulcerative colitis in 3). In the last 6 cases, although no liver biopsy was obtained, clinical evidence of liver disease was present.

There is no experimental or clinical explanation for this, but the assumption made by Turnberg and Grahame (281) that the cirrhotic liver fails to catabolize secretin, causing a higher effective dose, is intriguing. Gross et al. (100) also reported abnormally high volumes in patients with parenchymatous diseases of the liver, and we have made a similar observation in individual patients.

11
Duodenal Drainage (Cholecystokinin Biliary Drainage)

Although they are obviously not cytological in nature, the concurrent search for cholesterol crystals and bilirubinate pigment is part of the diagnostic usefulness of the duodenal drainage; hence a brief discussion of this subject is included.

The collection of biliary secretions through duodenal drainage was introduced by Lyon (167) in 1919, based upon Meltzer's (179) theory that relaxation of the ampulla of Vater would result in contraction of the gallbladder, with discharge of bile into the duodenum. This effect was induced by instilling a solution of magnesium sulfate into the duodenum through a gastroduodenal tube, introduced to the level of the third portion of the duodenum. Within a few minutes, a light golden yellow bile appeared from the common duct and was collected as the A fraction. A darker and more viscous fraction began to appear in 10 to 15 min and was collected as B bile or gallbladder bile. Finally, a thin light yellow bile, designated the C fraction, issued from the hepatic ducts and liver.

On microscopic examination of the sediment, cholesterol crystals and calcium bilirubinate granules were the first organized elements recognized and believed to have pathologic significance. The cholesterol crystals were described as thin colorless, transparent crystals with parallel edges, often having a notched corner (167, 168). The presence of more than a few cholesterol crystals soon was accepted as strongly suggestive of cholelithiasis, cholecystitis, or cholesterolosis, particularly if the crystals were present in clumps (28, 68, 91, 125, 127, 129, 155, 169, 215, 226, 228, 236, 237, 258, 295).

Calcium bilirubinate granules were described as finely granular precipitate, varying in color from pale golden yellow to bright orange. Anything more than very small amounts of calcium bilirubinate granules was considered abnormal and, in the absence of obstructive jaundice, strongly suggestive of cholelithiasis or cholecystitis or both (28, 127, 129, 168, 215, 226, 236, 237, 263). The presence of both cholesterol crystals and calcium bilirubinate granules was considered by almost all workers to indicate gallstone formation. However, the presence of these elements in the absence of biliary tree disease subsequently was reported in viral hepatitis (128, 152), in other hepatocellular causes of jaundice (28, 55, 129, 258), and in patients with hemolytic anemias (254).

The present study was undertaken to ascertain the clinical value of the search for cholesterol crystals and calcium bilirubinate granules in the biliary secretions obtained by duodenal drainage after stimulation with cholecystokinin.

Material and Methods

Our technique of duodenal intubation has been described in chapter 3. One Ivy-dog unit per kg body weight of Cecekin, diluted 1 to 10, is injected intravenously up to a maximum of 75 units. Its action is immediate, and in about 10 to 15 min B bile usually is collected in sufficient amount. All collected bile is centrifuged at 5,000 rpm for 20 min, and the sediment is examined for crystals and granules, usually by light microscopy, but more easily by phase microscopy.

During the period 1 January 1962 to 31 December 1969, 184 patients were studied. Adequate documentation and followup were possible in 178 cases.

Results

The results of the entire series are given in table 11.1; the percentage distribution of crystals and granules for each of the stated groups of diseases also is shown in table 11.1. In group I, patients with established disease of the biliary tract, 77% of 48 patients had cholesterol crystals or calcium bilirubinate granules or both. In group II, patients with disease of the liver or pancreas, including cirrhosis, pancreatitis, and pancreatic carcinoma, 40% of 42 patients had calcium bilirubinate granules. However, *none* of the patients of group II had cholesterol crystals, even in the presence of jaundice. In group III, including various diseases or states such as irritable digestive tract (68 patients), "postcholecystectomy syndrome" without demonstrable organic cause (7 patients), and miscellaneous (13 patients: 2 cases each of colonic diverticulitis, duodenal ulcer, gastrointestinal bleeding of undetermined origin, hiatus hernia; 1 case each of aortic aneurysm, amebic abscess of right kidney, angina pectoris, tropical sprue, and regional enteritis), 10% had calcium bilirubinate in the duodenal drainage, and 1 patient (with postcholecystectomy syndrome) had cholesterol crystals and calcium bilirubinate.

The correlation between the finding in 61 cases of cholesterol crystals or calcium bilirubinate granules or both and the groups of diseases is shown in table 11.2. The most striking figure is the one for cholesterol crystals: in 21 of the total of 22 patients, established disease

Material and Results at the
University of Chicago

TABLE 11.1

RESULTS OF DUODENAL DRAINAGE IN 178 PATIENTS

Disease Group	No. of Patients	Positive Findings [a] No.	%
Group I. Biliary tree diseases			
Cholecystitis, cholelithiasis, or both	40	32	
Postcholecystectomy syndrome with organic cause (stone, stricture, infection)	8	5	
Subtotal	48	37	77%
Group II. Diseases of liver or pancreas			
Cirrhosis	11	6	
Pericholangitis	1	1	
Hepatitis, viral	5	2	
Pancreatic carcinoma	16	3	
Carcinoma of common bile duct	1	1	
Chronic relapsing pancreatitis	8	3	
Subtotal	42	16	40%
Group III. Patients without organic hepatobiliary or pancreatic disease ("controls")			
Functional bowel distress	68	1	
Postcholecystectomy syndrome without organic cause	7	1	
Miscellaneous diseases	13	6	
Subtotal	88	8	10%
TOTAL	178	61	

[a] Calcium bilirubinate granules or cholesterol crystals or both. For more details see table 11.2. In 10 other patients no B bile was obtained, all patients being jaundiced. Four patients had carcinoma of the head of the pancreas, 3 had common duct stone, and 3 had cirrhosis.

TABLE 11.2

DISTRIBUTION OF 61 POSITIVE DUODENAL DRAINAGES
BY DISEASE GROUPS

Finding	No. of Patients	Group I No.	%	Group II No.	%	Group III No.	%
Cholesterol crystals [a]	22	21	(95.5)	0	(−)	1	(4.5) [a]
Calcium bilirubinate granules only	39	16	(41)	16	(41)	7	(18)
	61	37	(60)	16	(26.6)	8	(13.4)

NOTE: See table 11.1 for breakdown of diseases by group.
[a] With accompanying calcium bilirubinate granules. This patient had a postcholecystectomy syndrome without organic cause demonstrated, but was not surgically reexplored.

of the biliary tract was present (group I). The only false-positive was in a patient with postcholecystectomy syndrome in whom no organic disease was demonstrable. Table 11.2 also indicates the low specificity of the

TABLE 11.3

CORRELATION BETWEEN ORAL CHOLECYSTOGRAPHY AND RESULTS OF
DUODENAL DRAINAGE IN CHOLECYSTITIS, CHOLELITHIASIS, OR BOTH

	No. of Cases	Positive	Duodenal Drainage Calcium Bilirubinate Plus Cholesterol Crystals	Calcium Bilirubinate Only	Negative
X rays diagnostic	22	17	10	7	5
X rays non-diagnostic [a]	18	15	11	4	3
Total	40	32	21	11	8

NOTE: N = 40.
[a] Patients with normal oral cholecystogram; faint visualization without stone; no visualization in presence of 3.0 mg% of total serum bilirubin or more.

finding of calcium bilirubinate granules, since only 41% of the cases found were in group I.

These observations suggest that the search for cholesterol crystals and calcium bilirubinate granules in the bile is a useful complementary procedure to the radiographic and cytologic investigation of the biliary tree. The finding of cholesterol crystals is particularly helpful and is highly suggestive of cholecystitis or gallstones or both (table 11.3). In the 40 patients with cholecystitis, cholelithiasis, or both, the oral cholecystogram was diagnostic in 22 cases, but was of limited clinical help in 18 instances, owing to the finding of a normal cholecystogram, faint visualization of the gallbladder without demonstration of stones, or complete nonvisualization in the presence of a total serum bilirubin in excess of 3.0 mg%. In these 18 patients, the duodenal drainage was positive in 15 instances and was of critical value in the 11 cases with cholesterol crystals. The main indication for the test, therefore, is the investigation of patients with suspected cholelithiasis who have nondiagnostic roentgenographic studies.

Our results [1] are in close agreement with the experience of Bockus (26), who, utilizing the magnesium sulfate technique of biliary drainage, has correlated the presence of cholesterol crystals and calcium bilirubinate pigment with cholelithiasis in approximately 95% of patients.

1. The collaboration of Dr. Duane W. Taebel in this study is gratefully acknowledged.

12
Colonic Cytology

The prognosis in carcinoma of the colon and rectum remains poor despite improved surgical techniques, although survival rates in *resectable* lesions are favorable. Too frequently the tumor is far advanced when diagnosed, a continuing problem even though at least 50% of these tumors are within the reach of the examining finger and approximately two-thirds are accessible to the sigmoidoscope. Adequate roentgenographic examination of the colon should disclose the remaining one-third. The further development of fiberoptic colonoscopy, permitting the direct examination of the descending colon, transverse colon, and ascending colon and sigmoid, should eventually provide an additional diagnostic approach. The delays in diagnosis usually are due to the patient's disregard of "early symptoms" and to the physician's frequent omission of those simple diagnostic measures.

Exfoliative cytology is of little practical usefulness when lesions are within the reach of the sigmoidoscope, but occasionally this technique is of value in evaluating lesions beyond the sigmoidoscope. Unfortunately, colon cytology at present remains time-consuming and cumbersome and can be somewhat strenuous for the patient. Because of these considerations, colonic cytology remains of little clinical usefulness. The recent development of fiberoptic colonoscopes may change this, if it can be demonstrated that cytology and biopsy with this instrument are of value in patients with lesions beyond the reach of the conventional sigmoidoscope (figs. 12.1, 12.2), and the instrument may facilitate direct-vision cytology, as in the stomach.

The following review of our experience with colonic cytology reveals the relatively high accuracy of the method and its usefulness in the study of certain conditions, such as ulcerative colitis.

Material

The initial experience with colonic cytology in this laboratory was reviewed in 1955 by Galambos and Klayman (80) and in 1964 by Raskin (223), covering the period from April 1955 to December 1961 (series I). From January 1962 to December 1968, 135 additional patients were studied by the same technique (series II).

After the exclusion of patients with incomplete followup (less than eighteen months) or inadequate clinical or histologic data, 704 patients were available for the present study, accounting for 737 procedures. We again emphasize our method of reporting: patients with more than one examination in whom the initial test was reported unsatisfactory, but in whom a repeat examination in the next few days proved to be positive or negative, are listed as positive or negative as determined in the second study. When repeat examinations were done more than two weeks apart, the first evaluation is included in the analysis, regardless of the result of the repeat examination.

The group of 704 patients includes 112 with proved malignant tumors and 592 considered free of cancer by followup or histologic data or both.

Results

Accuracy

The results are condensed in table 12.1. Of the 112 malignant tumors 87 were correctly diagnosed, a sensitivity of 77.6%. Eighteen tumors were reported as negative by cytology, and 7 had unsatisfactory tests that for various reasons were not repeated.

The 592 patients free of cancer were correctly diagnosed as negative in 550 instances, 38 had unsatisfactory tests not repeated, and 4 had positive cytology (false-positive). These 4 patients represent 0.7% of the total number of patients with negative followup and 4.4% of the positive cytology reports. The specificity of the positive report, therefore, is of the order of 96%.

TABLE 12.1

DIAGNOSTIC ACCURACY OF COLONIC CYTOLOGY:
SALINE ENEMAS METHOD

Lesion	No. of Patients	Positive Cytology	Positive Report Analysis	Negative Cytology	Unsatisfactory
Clinically benign lesion or normal colon			*Specificity*		
Series I [a]	475	2	—	438	35
Series II	117	2	—	112	3
Total	592	4	95.6%	550	38
Proved malignant tumors			*Sensitivity*		
Series I [a]	94	70	—	17	7
Series II	18	17	—	1	—
Total	112	87	77.6%	18	7

NOTE: University of Chicago series; 704 patients.
[a] Data of Raskin et al. (223).

Material and Results at the University of Chicago

Correlation between the Cytologic and Histopathologic Findings

All the malignant tumors were adenocarcinomas, mostly well differentiated and with abundant mucus production. In 5 cases the lesion was a "malignant villous adenoma" or, more correctly, cancer arising in a villous adenoma. In 3 instances the appearance was of a small polypoid carcinoma without invasion of the muscularis mucosae ("carcinoma in situ"). All patients with positive cytology presented an adenocarcinoma type of cytological picture, except for 5 cases presenting an anaplastic type of malignancy. This finding is not disturbing, because carcinoma of the colon beyond the reach of the rectosigmoidoscope almost invariably is adenocarcinoma. Malignant lymphoma of the colon was not encountered.

Comments and Review of the Literature

Accuracy of Cytology

Exfoliative cytology by colonic washings of lesions beyond the search of the rectosigmoidoscope is reasonably accurate but is not easily performed. The procedure is time-consuming and is unsatisfactory in approximately 7% of attempts. The sensitivity of 77.6% in the presence of a malignant tumor is rewarding, and methods of simplifying the procedure and diminishing the unsatisfactory procedures while maintaining or even improving the sensitivity should be sought.

Very few other laboratories have reported the use of colonic washings similar to our technique; Thabet and Knoerschild (275–77), who use millepore filtration instead of centrifugation, recorded 27 positive cytodiagnoses in a series of 46 cases of colon carcinoma, and Miller et al. (183) noted 13 positive cytodiagnoses in 17 cases of colon carcinoma. Unfortunately, Thabet and Knoerschild reported about 20% unsatisfactory procedures; and in the series described by Miller et al. as many as 24% of positive reports originated in clinically benign situations. The Papanicolaou classification in the reporting was used by both groups, and class III cases were computed with the positive reports by Thabet and Knoerschild, a practice which we feel should be abandoned.

Errors in Cytology

In 4 patients, the followup failed to reveal cancer of the colon, but the cytodiagnosis had been positive for malignant cells (false-positive cases). They represent 0.7% of the total number of benign cases and 4.4% of the positive cytology reports.

The first error was in a patient with diverticulosis and lymphoma of the transverse colon. The second instance was that of an elderly female who had a small polypoid lesion approximately 33 cm above the anal ring, barely reached by the biopsy forceps; the fragment of tissue was considered suspicious of carcinoma. Since the X rays were negative, a cytologic procedure was performed and a few malignant-looking cells were obtained. A second sigmoidoscopic examination made in an effort to obtain additional confirmatory biopsies failed to disclose a lesion up to a level of 30 cm. The patient was operated upon several weeks later and no tumor or neoplasm was found. Raskin (223) concluded that the patient may have had a carcinoma in situ in a polyp which subsequently became necrotic and sloughed. The third instance was that of a young female with recent onset of diarrhea. The clinical picture, in retrospect, was of a probable infectious diarrhea. The episode was self-limited and the patient is well and free of colonic symptoms six years later. The fourth patient had diverticulitis of the sigmoid colon. He responded to medical therapy. A repeat cytological examination, one week after the clinical remission, did not reveal any suspicious or malignant cells. The patient is well and free of symptoms four years later.

In an early report from this laboratory (222), a false-positive report was obtained in a patient with an adenomatous polyp that yielded malignant-appearing cells, but histology failed to reveal tumor. One year later, the remaining portions of the polyp were resected and carcinoma in situ was found (223).

Of 112 carcinomas beyond proctoscopic range, 18 were negative (about 16%) and 7 (about 6%) had unsatisfactory tests which were not repeated. Raskin (223) commented on the decrease in accuracy that followed the substitution of a fine-mesh strainer for a coarse one, observed in series I, comparison being made with an earlier report (222) from the same laboratory; in series II a coarse-mesh strainer was reintroduced, with significantly better results.

In 48 instances (about 7% of the total number of procedures) the test was considered unsatisfactory because of heavy fecal contamination, poor cell preservation, scarcity of diagnostic cells, or a combination of these factors; 7 of these were patients with carcinoma of the colon.

Safety

The safety record of the procedure is excellent. The only serious accident was reported by Raskin (223); a large solitary diverticulum just below the level of a sigmoid stricture was perforated by the tip of the Ewald tube.

Cell Collection Methods

The method used in our laboratory and described in detail in chapter 3 has been most accurate and is associated with less sampling error in lesions beyond the reach of the sigmoidoscope. However, it is a very time-consuming procedure and has not found very large acceptance, judging by the paucity of reports using the same technique (46, 183, 275–77).

More recently, Vacca and deLuca (286) and Miller et al. (183) have suggested a simplification of the technique utilizing the flecks of mucus, tissue, or blood trapped by a fine-mesh strainer as the source of diagnostic cells, instead of centrifuging the filtered fluid. We should note parenthetically that we collect and smear any fleck of blood-tinged mucus trapped by the coarse-mesh strainer. Actually, the most cumbersome and time-consuming step is the preparation of the patient.

Vacca and his colleagues prepared the patient on the day before examination by the use of a cathartic and used a single cleansing diagnostic enema (about 2,000 ml of saline solution). The returns from this enema then were strained and mucus particles were selected for smearing. This technique takes less time, but the accuracy rate of 60% (19 positive reports in 35 colonic cancers) is disappointing.

Knoerschild (143), Cameron (45, 46), and Thabet (276, 277) at Ohio State University Medical Center developed the millepore filtration method for colonic cytology, and have attempted a modified mass screening program. In one study of rectal mucosa smears obtained from 17,000 patients (276), they reported 79% diagnostic accuracy in 132 visible carcinomas of the colon but a disappointing 5% in the 96 patients in whom the lesion was beyond the range of the proctoscope. Thus, routine rectal cytologic smears seem to be of little value in diagnosing nonvisible lesions of the large bowel.

A technique utilizing differences in specific gravity between feces and exfoliated cells has been developed by Hampton, Bacon, and Myer (193). The fecal particles are separated from the exfoliated cells by a silicone barrier at the time of centrifugation. This approach is intriguing and should be confirmed by additional studies.

Another method for collecting cells uses silicone foam, as suggested by Spjut, Cook, and Margolis (265). A silicone foam cast of the left side of the colon can be obtained by the in vivo polymerization of the plastic. A soft pliable mold or cast of the colon is expelled in minutes to hours, and any area of indentation made by tumor, polyp, or stricture is subsequently irrigated and examined for malignant cells. Twelve of 13 persons with colonic carcinomas were reported by the cytologists as "suspicious" of carcinoma or as positive.

Cytology of Lesions within the Reach of the Proctosigmoidoscope

The cytologic study of lesions within reach of the proctosigmoidoscope usually is reserved for research or special studies (5, 12, 16, 23, 79, 81, 142, 164, 192–94, 297). Such lesions obviously should be biopsied, and frequently they are removed in toto.

In 1951, Loeb and Scapier (164) described a double pump instrument for irrigation of the rectosigmoid area (using saline solution) during proctosigmoidoscopy, especially designed for tumors of the left side of the colon. This technique was employed most extensively by Bader and Papanicolaou (12), with reasonably good results, but the use of class III reporting and the emphasis on the diagnosis of polyps by cytology impaired the overall accuracy of the method. Galambos (79, 81), in this laboratory, employed a similar device for studying the rectal mucosa cytology of patients with chronic ulcerative colitis. Oakland (192–94) reported the use of rectal washings, even in lesions within range of the proctosigmoidoscope, on the basis that a biopsy may be taken at a point some inches distal to the important lesion and thus be inconclusive.

Ayre (11), in 1959, described his cytology brush for use in colonic lesions up to the splenic flexure, under fluoroscopic control. The largest series reported with this cell collection method was that of Heidenreich (106) in 1961, with 300 patients. The somewhat high rate of false-positive reports (5%) complicates interpretation of the series.

**Material and Results at the
University of Chicago**

Exfoliative Cytology in Chronic Ulcerative Colitis

The increased incidence of carcinoma in association with chronic ulcerative colitis is well documented (59, 93, 114). Also, pronounced epithelial atypias have been described in chronic ulcerative colitis, and their "premalignant" nature has been emphasized by Morson and Pang (187). Furthermore, the symptoms of carcinoma of the colon frequently mimic simple exacerbation of colitis, and the radiological diagnosis of malignant lesions in the ulcerative colitis colon is not uniformly easy (70). To further complicate the diagnostic problem, the routine periodical radiologic examinations of patients with chronic ulcerative colitis is not devoid of risks, including severe recurrences of the colitis. Galambos et al. (81), in a previous study from this laboratory, described attempts to use exfoliative cytology for the diagnosis of colonic cancer in chronic ulcerative colitis. These observations demonstrated the presence of several types of cells in the material obtained by both colonic washings and rectal irrigation in patients with chronic ulcerative colitis. Most disturbing, in addition to obviously benign cells ("bland" and "active" cells), in 4 cases there were malignant-appearing cells in the absence of any clinical or histological evidence of carcinoma. These malignant-appearing cells were seen only in the active phase.

In 3 other patients, "lymphoma" cells were recovered. No details were given on the type of lymphoma cells. No malignant lymphoma was clinically detected in the followup, but lymphoreticular hyperplasia probably was present (2 patients had previous subtotal colectomies and I had had an "anal mass" removed).

Cytochemical methods for the demonstration of enzymes such as succinic dehydrogenase and DPN diaphorase failed to reveal significant differences between colonic cells of patients with chronic ulcerative colitis and malignant cells of patients with carcinoma of the colon (13).

Anthonisen and Riis (5) have shown an increased eosinophil count in colonic secretions, studied by a touch preparation, in patients with ulcerative colitis. The significance of this finding, in their opinion, is mainly diagnostic. Similar observations were made by Boddington and Truelove (29).

In the present series, 63 patients with chronic ulcerative colitis were studied by the colonic washing method. The previously described "active" and "bland" cells again were demonstrated in most instances. In 2 cases, malignant-appearing cells were recovered and in a third patient larger and undifferentiated lymphoid cells were abundantly present. The followup has not revealed malignant tumor in any of the 3 individuals.

In 5 additional patients, malignant cells were recovered and adenocarcinoma of the colon complicating ulcerative colitis was found at surgery. Morphologically, we could not detect any difference between the cells of these 5 cases and the cells of the 2 cases in whom cancer has not been found. These cells probably are derived from in situ carcinomas and only a prolonged followup may unravel the true sequence of events regarding malignant transformation of the colonic mucosa in ulcerative colitis, a study that should be made.

Similar cellular atypias in scrapings of the rectal mucosa from patients with ulcerative colitis have been described by Boddington and Truelove (29). They also emphasized the morphological similarities between the most atypical cells and malignant cells.

At present, a study is being conducted in our Gastroenterology Section (by Dr. J. B. Kirsner and others) to further delineate the extent and morphology of the atypical epithelial hyperplasias and carcinoma in situ ("premalignant changes" of Morson) in ulcerative colitis.

Part 4

Atlas of Cell Morphology in the Gastrointestinal Tract

13
Cytologic Criteria of Malignancy

The subject of criteria of malignancy in exfoliative cytology is most important. However, the cytologist must emphasize that no single morphological criterion per se is pathognomonic for malignancy. Rather, a combination of criteria, evaluated on the basis of previous experience, is utilized for the final evaluation. In this sense, the cytological report remains subjective. However, the decision of an experienced cytopathologist usually is correct, in the sense that the histopathologist finds a malignant tumor when the cytological report is positive for malignant cells and does not find a neoplasm when the cytological report is negative for malignant cells. Very occasionally, the histopathologist finds a malignant tumor overlooked by the cytopathologist (usually on the basis of poor sampling rather than misinterpretation of adequate diagnostic material). Also occasionally, the histopathologist finds no tumor in an area examined by the cytopathologist and reported as positive for malignant cells. The cause of this discrepancy usually is the presence of atypical epithelium. In the gastrointestinal tract, healing peptic ulcers, chronic ulcerative colitis, and polyps with atypical epithelial changes are the most common conditions in this category. The two latter conditions probably are either premalignant or already may represent in situ carcinoma. Further studies are needed to better understand this group of disorders. In the subsequent paragraphs the usual morphological criteria for malignancy (table 13.1) and their relative importance in exfoliative cytology of the gastrointestinal tract are discussed.

Nuclear Changes

Nuclear Enlargement: Anisonucleosis

An increased interphase nuclear volume (absolute nuclear enlargement) is a regular finding in almost every malignant tumor. Usually the cytoplasm does not enlarge in the same proportion, and the result is an increased nuclear-cytoplasmic index (relative nuclear enlargement).

However, the same finding is frequent in almost all types of cell proliferation (e.g., adenomas or healing of ulcerative lesions), and is a regular effect of irradiation (38). It is often seen in epithelial cells (as well as in bone marrow cells) of patients with vitamin B_{12} or folic acid deficiency (30, 82, 96, 98, 177, 190, 266). An important differential point in malignant tumors is the

frequent finding of large and small cells side by side (anisokaryosis and anisocytosis). In benign conditions such findings are rare; the nuclear enlargement is more regular and the cell population is more homogeneous.

Saito et al. (248) measured the maximum diameter of nuclei in smears prepared by direct scraping or surgically resected specimens of gastric mucosa, both from the tumor itself and from the surrounding areas.

TABLE 13.1

CYTOLOGIC CRITERIA OF MALIGNANCY

Nuclear Changes
  Nuclear enlargement and anisonucleosis
  Increase and abnormality in the chromatin content
  Nuclear pleomorphism
  Enlarged or abnormal nucleoli
  Multinucleation associated with nuclear atypia
  Abnormal mitotic figures
  Degenerative changes
Cytoplasmic Changes
  Pronounced eosinophilia
  Cytoplasmic inclusions
  "Cannibalism"
  Pigment granules
  Atypical vacuolation
Changes of the Cell as a Whole
  Changes in cell size and shape
Changes in the Interrelationship between the Cells
  Tendency to exfoliate as isolated single cells
  Irregular grouping with nuclear crowding and loss of defined cell limits
  Characteristic patterns: rosette, palisade

Under phase-contrast microscopy, the maximum diameter of nonmalignant gastric epithelial cells ranged between 5 μ and 17 μ, averaging 10.5 μ, whereas that of cancer cells varied between 7 μ and 30 μ, the vast majority measuring 14 μ or more. There was considerable overlap between the two curves of distribution, but the nonmalignant cells had a much narrower distribution.

Each tumor usually has a predominant nuclear size (stemline), generally larger than the corresponding normal tissue. The nuclear enlargement is usually attributed to the hyperploidy so frequently found in malignant tumors. Miles and Koss (182) demonstrated that in heterotransplanted human tumors the nuclear area correlated to some extent with the number and total length of chromosomes, but the relationship was not uniformly definite. Atkin (9), using squash preparations, found each tumor to have a predominant nuclear size that correlated well with the karyotype as well as with the DNA content (8). It should also be noted that extreme degrees of hyperploidy seldom are found in solid tumors, in contrast to cancer cells in pleural or ascitic fluid, which frequently are characterized by high degrees of hyperploidy.

Increase and Abnormality in the Chromatin Content

Abnormal chromatin structure, including hyperchromatism and abnormal centers, frequently is seen in smears stained by the Papanicolaou method and is often quoted as the most reliable criterion of malignancy. However, such changes may represent varying degrees of degeneration and artifacts caused by delays in fixation during cell collection. They are much less obvious in direct-vision smears, where there usually is minimal degeneration and the fixation process is immediate and very rapid. It is also the experience of cytologists using MGG stained smears that such findings are never conspicuous. Similarly, the extreme degree of chromatin abnormality is seen in hematoxylin and eosin stained sections. Thus, the pronounced marginal condensation of chromatin (sometimes creating the false impression of marked thickening of the nuclear membrane) which is often impressive in sections and in Papanicolaou stained smears is hardly ever seen in dry-fixed smears or in direct-vision smears. A somewhat intermediate picture is observed in the fine structure (X 25,000) of nuclei fixed by glutaraldehyde and stained by uranyl ions; even normal nuclei show marginal condensation of chromatin (69).

The quantitative (cytophotometry) determination of DNA content and variation is an important aspect of this problem, because it is one of the bases for automated cytodiagnosis. In a study by Sandritter, Carl, and Ritter (249), at least 13% of the cells of all 30 tested tumors (including 9 tumors of the digestive system) had DNA content above the triploid range.

The finding of hypochromatic nuclei is not rare in gastric washings, in our experience, and may be the expression of the poor cell preservation. Allen and Fullmer (2) reported one case of gastric carcinoma in which almost all cells had very hypochromatic nuclei; the pictures illustrating their report demonstrate poorly preserved cells.

Nuclear Pleomorphism

Nuclear pleomorphism has been recognized as a distinctive feature of malignant tumors since the time of Virchow. It is very difficult to find two nuclei which are precisely similar. The occurrence of *monomorphism,* however, is quite spectacular in some cases. Söderström (264) stressed that "in normal cell populations there is some degree of anisokaryosis," and it has been shown by Jacobj (123) that "in normal cell populations this variation in nuclear size is not continuous; there are a few type classes of nuclei with respect to volume, within each class of nuclei are grossly of equal size, and the numerical relation between the different volume classes is a simple doubling (1–2–4, etc.)."

The frequent finding of spectacular types of bizarre nuclei is one reason why anaplastic tumors are more easily recognized cytologically than are well-differentiated tumors. Again, chronic ulcerative colitis is an example of a nonmalignant condition where bizarre nuclei shapes are occasionally seen. Bizarre nuclei probably represent a sort of by-product of all types of cell proliferation in adverse conditions—for example, the formation of giant cells with very bizarre nuclei during radiation therapy of tumors. It is interesting to note that in one patient who had had mild gastric irradiation of adjunctive therapy for peptic ulcer, rather abnormal-looking cells were observed in the gastric washing.

Dwarf cells are seen occasionally, especially in squamous cell carcinoma. They usually are frequent in large and necrotic tumors, an observation also made by authors dealing with bronchogenic carcinoma (151).

Enlarged or Abnormal Nucleoli

Söderström (264) analyzes this criterion in an excellent manner: "Large nucleoli are found in all types of proliferation." Caspersson and Santesson (51) distinguished, in malignant cell populations, cells with cytoplasm rich in RNA [1] and rather small nucleoli (A cells), and cells with large nucleoli and a cytoplasm poor in RNA (B cells), representing different types of metabolic activity. Examples of this dualism are often seen in exfoliative cytology.

"Nucleoli of extreme dimensions are especially important in the diagnosis of otherwise well differentiated malignant tumors. Nucleoli of a comparable size may also be seen in Reed-Sternberg cells." Sometimes the identification of a small nucleolus is difficult because of the increased nucleolus-associated chromatin content

---

1. Deeply basophilic with the MGG stain.

that obscures it. "On the other hand, the absence of visible nucleoli does not constitute evidence against malignancy; this is instead a typical feature of some malignant tumor cells, especially in tumors with a dominant stem line of small rather uniform cells (264)."

Medak et al. (178) have described oral lesions in pemphigus vulgaris, in which the epithelial cells had very large and irregular nucleoli, and Forni, Koss, and Geller (73), studying the effects of cyclophosphamide on bladder epithelial cells, demonstrated large irregular nucleoli, emphasizing the nonspecific nature of this cytological finding.

In chapter 7 we commented upon the finding of very large nucleoli in cells from benign gastric ulcers.

Multinucleation and Nuclear Lobulation Associated with Nuclear Atypia

The presence of multiple nuclei in the same cell is fairly frequent in malignant tumor; however, it is not a specific finding. Other types of abnormal epithelial proliferation, such as in the healing of benign peptic ulcer, use of cyclophosphamide (73), or irradiation (38), also are associated with this change. However, the malignant multinucleated cell usually manifests at the same time marked nuclear pleomorphism, and benign conditions have less pleomorphic nuclei. In this context, it should be noted that blistering and vesicular diseases of the oral epithelium are particularly prone to exfoliate multinucleated atypical cells (38, 178), and it is always useful to inspect the oral cavity before proceeding with gastrointestinal intubation for exfoliative cytology.

Sometimes it is difficult to decide if the cell manifests multinucleation or multilobulation. Both phenomena are expressions of abnormal cell proliferation. That multilobulation (and probably nuclear fragmentation also) is a fairly frequent phenomenon has been demonstrated by several studies using electron microscopy, and is frequently mentioned by cytologists using air-dried smears that produce a "flatter" picture of the cell (264).

Nuclear lobulation is seen frequently in malignant cells (76, 162) and, at least in some cases, it may represent a derangement in cell growth and in messenger RNA transfer to the cytoplasm (76). How giant multinucleate cells are formed is not entirely clear. The most accepted mechanism is by incomplete cytokinesis, but the intriguing possibility that in some cases they form by coalescence of cells connected by bridges (actually tubules) has been raised (57); this also could explain the synchronous mitotic activity occasionally seen in malignant tumors.

A remarkable observation is that each lobule or segment of the giant cells often is provided with a large single nucleolus or a macrochromocenter (22, 76).

Lobulation is not specific to tumor cells; it can be seen in the segmentation of megakaryocyte nuclei and the nuclear segmentation in mesothelial and endothelial cells (262).

Free nuclear fragments within the cytoplasm are often seen in malignant cells. In some cases the fragments are numerous and unequal in size, and may simply represent a disorganized splitting of the nuclei in dying cells (especially in some giant cells seen after radiation therapy) (264). The findings of multiple small necrotic cells and of prominent karyorrhexis are rather common in malignant lymphomas (see chap. 15) but are seen occasionally in carcinomas (18).

Free nuclear fragments have a high value as signs of malignancy; they are rarely seen in cells belonging to nonmalignant populations (264). The finding of nuclear protrusions, probably caused by a marker chromosome, has been reported in many gynecologic tumors (9). This abnormality is best demonstrated in squash or well-flattened preparations and is difficult to demonstrate with the usual Papanicolaou technique.

Radial segmentation of the nuclei is an interesting phenomenon which is present to a moderate degree in the majority of malignant tumors and is a very conspicuous feature in many of them, again best seen in air-dried preparations.

In the experience of Söderström (264), radial segmentation may appear simply as a number of shallow indentations in the margin of the nucleus, making its contour seem more or less polycyclic. The apparently two-dimensional view offered by smear preparations may conceal the fact that some of these indentations in reality are deep clefts through the nucleus, dividing it into separate segments; nuclear clefts have been noted frequently in electron microscopy; the indentations and clefts converge toward a certain point in the nuclear periphery, usually marked by a blunt impression.

Abnormal Mitotic Figures

The presence of obviously abnormal mitoses, such as a tripolar figure, is highly suggestive of malignancy. Unfortunately, they are exceedingly rare. Numerous mitoses are a good screening sign, but in direct-vision brushing specimens they must be interpreted very cautiously. Two of our false-positive diagnoses were made on the basis of the finding of numerous mitoses and cellular atypias. Both cases were proved to be healing peptic ulcers.

Abnormally high numbers of chromosomes are frequently seen in pleural or ascitic fluid preparations from metastatic gastrointestinal tumors.

Degenerative Changes (Vacuolation, Fading, or Resorption of the Nucleus)

The presence of degenerative changes, such as nuclear vacuolation, fading, or resorption, is a good screening sign of malignancy. They are much more common in malignant cells than in benign conditions. However, they are *not* diagnostic. Nuclear vacuolation probably is only an indication of cell death before fixation (151). The complete resorption of the nucleus is seen frequently in squamous cell carcinoma. The presence of multiple "ghost" cells, highly eosinophilic keratinized cytoplasmic spherules, is a good screening sign and usually indicates the presence of a necrotic squamous cell carcinoma.

Cytoplasmic Changes

Pronounced Eosinophilia

Squamous cell carcinomas usually are easy to recognize because of the peculiar hyaline and eosinophilic cytoplasm of keratinized cells that also have gross nuclear pleomorphism. In benign conditions, when the squamous cytoplasm is eosinophilic or keratinized or both, the nucleus is quite small and pyknotic.

The presence of small "ghost" eosinophilic cells devoid of nucleus has been commented upon earlier in this chapter.

Cytoplasmic Inclusions

Fat droplets are easily recognized in MGG stained smears but are difficult to identify in Papanicolaou stained smears. *Glycogen granules* are occasionally seen in malignant squamous cells. Various types of *inclusion bodies* or nuclear fragments are seen frequently, but are more difficult to interpret because they are also noted in benign inflammatory conditions.

"Cannibalism"

It is common to attribute to malignant cells the property of phagocytosis. However, most of these instances prob-

ably represent incomplete separation of daughter cells after division. The "bird's-eye" cell probably is the best example of this phenomenon. Truly phagocytized materials usually are quickly digested by the cell.

The presence of inflammatory cells, usually neutrophils, inside epithelial cells is seen in equal incidence in inflammation and neoplasia (benign and malignant tumors alike).

The presence of lymphocytes inside epithelial cells of the digestive tract is an interesting phenomenon (4) without relationship to neoplastic transformation. Discussion of its physiologic implications is beyond the scope of this review.

Pigment Granules

In one exceptional case of metastatic malignant melanoma of the stomach seen in this laboratory by Reed, Raskin, and Graff (225), there were abundant typical pigment granules.

Atypical Vacuolation

Large, Simple Mucinlike Vacuoles. The presence of typical signet-ring cells is very common in gastric carcinoma; only occasionally are they absent. The typical signet-ring cell is an isolated cell with a large cytoplasmic vacuole and well-demarcated limits ("walls") that pushes the nucleus to the periphery. The nucleus usually is quite abnormal, with one large nucleolus. PAS staining of the vacuole is strongly positive.

Multiple Small Vacuoles. Less commonly recognized, but of equal diagnostic importance, are isolated cells with multiple small cytoplasmic vacuoles and an atypical but not very pleomorphic nucleus. The cytoplasm, owing to the presence of multiple small vacuoles, has a foamy appearance, and such cells are called "foam cells." They are usually seen in conjunction with typical signet-ring cells, but in one patient they were the only evidence for malignancy (gastric adenocarcinoma). However, cytoplasmic vacuolation should be interpreted cautiously, because it is one of the most consistent irradiation effects on cells (38). Alkylating agents, such as cyclophosphamide, also produce cytoplasmic vacuolation, especially of the urinary tract epithelium (73). A foamy cytoplasm also is characteristic of histiocytes, obviously nonmalignant cells. These findings decrease the diagnostic value of "foam cells."

Changes of the Cell as a Whole

Changes in Cell Size and Shape

Cancer cells originating in the squamous epithelium of the esophagus always display a pronounced variation in cell size (anisocytosis). Adenocarcinoma cells from the other areas of the gastrointestinal tract exhibit a lesser degree of anisocytosis. Considerable variation from normal shape also is a common characteristic of squamous cell carcinomas, the more typical being the so-called *tadpole cell* and the *fiber cell*. Again, adenocarcinomas exhibit less variation than the squamous cell carcinomas.

The relative areas of the nucleus and of the cytoplasm, together with the total extinction of the cytoplasm, have been utilized in a computerized self-learning program as descriptors for cell identification (TICAS) with very high accuracy, emphasizing the real differences between cancer and benign cells of the same tissue. However, the complexity of this index has not permitted their quantitative assessment thus far (293).

Interrelationship between the Cells

The finding of *single, isolated* well-preserved cells is very rare in exfoliative cytology of the normal gastro-intestinal tract distal to the cardioesophageal junction. This finding per se is a good screening sign for malignancy. Sometimes the only evidence for cancer is the finding of a few signet-ring or "foam" cells (229), as was explained in the previous section, resulting from the decreased adhesiveness between cancer cells (56, 83). This abnormality is attributed chiefly to a reduced calcium content in the intercellular spaces.

The finding of large groups of cells with nuclear crowding and loss of well-defined cell limits is frequent in anaplastic tumors, but in this situation the degree of nuclear pleomorphism is the more important criterion. The problem of the "cannibalism" has been commented upon earlier.

The cells of malignant lymphoma always are found as isolated cells and never form cohesive groups (see chap. 15 for discussion of the cytology of malignant lymphomas of the stomach).

The finding of a characteristic pattern, such as the rosette form, is rare in washing cytology, but is seen occasionally in direct-vision brushing specimens or in pleural or ascitic fluid specimens.

14

Morphology of Benign and Malignant Exfoliated Cells of the Gastrointestinal Mucosa

The morphology of the epithelial cells of the gastrointestinal tract, both the benign and the malignant counterparts, has been reviewed in detail in several publications from this laboratory (79, 81, 208, 216, 242). In the following pages, an iconographic atlas of the more characteristic findings in our experience is offered. To avoid repetition and to save space, the text explains each figure, and the captions for the figures identify them.

The color pictures all were taken (except when otherwise noted) with a Leitz Laborlux microscope, equipped with an Ipso photographic attachment, using Kodachrome Type Professional II A. From such transparencies the color plates were made. The enlargements noted in the captions always refer to the original enlargement given by the ocular-objective combination of the microscope. The reader should remember that the Ipso attachment itself has an enlargement factor of 1.25 and the final printed picture also is an enlargement of the original 35 mm transparency. However, these two enlargements are constant and apply to all pictures, making the comparison between pictures accurate and meaningful.

Finally, the pictures for ideal analysis should be viewed with a light source (tungsten) with approximately 3,200 K color temperature. Other light sources, such as ordinary fluorescent light, give various color distortions. However, this is not particularly critical because of the practical impossibility of reproducing exactly the original color balance of the specimen.

I. Morphology of the Cells Stained by the Papanicolaou Method

Esophagus

Normal Esophagus

Histology. The esophageal mucosa is composed of a stratified noncornifying squamous epithelium, with three main zones: (a) superficial, (b) intermediate or parabasal, and (c) basal. The lamina propria consists of loose connective tissue, throughout which numerous lymphocytes are scattered. At the junction with the cardia of the stomach, there is an abrupt transition to a simple columnar epithelium.

Cytology. The cells of the *superficial* layers of the epithelium (figs. 14.1 to 14.4) are characterized by an abundant polygonal cytoplasm and one small, occasionally pyknotic, nucleus. The cytoplasm may contain a small number of keratohyalin granules but does not undergo cornification. The nucleus is oval, and its chromatin content is evenly distributed in small granules. Occasionally the sex-chromatin Barr's body may be identified. The cells are exfoliated singly or in large sheets. The characteristic "pearl" formation (fig. 14.4) of concentrically arranged cells may be seen.

The cells of the *intermediate* layer of the epithelium (fig. 14.5) are characterized by a relatively larger vesicular nucleus (occasionally binucleated cells are seen), absence of cytoplasmic keratohyalin granules, and a polygonal or oval cell shape. In direct-vision brushing material, they are frequent and are shed singly or in large sheets.

The *basal* cells (fig. 14.6) have large nuclei and scanty cytoplasm. The nucleus frequently is hyperchromatic and contains a large nucleolus. The presence of basal cells results from vigorous brushing or exfoliation from an eroded lesion. Again, they may exfoliate singly or in sheets. Isolated basal cells should not be confused with malignant cells, and the finding of similar cells in flat sheets is an important clue to their benign nature. Sometimes, as is illustrated in fig. 14.6, the cells are clustered and there is considerable overlapping of nuclei. Care should be taken not to confuse such groups with malignant cells. Mitoses are relatively frequent in large sheets of basal cells.

Benign Lesions of the Esophagus

Esophagitis. Especially in its chronic ulcerative type, this lesion exfoliates intermediate or basal cells singly or in sheets. As was stated earlier, sometimes the basal cells are difficult to differentiate from malignant cells. The presence of inflammatory cells in the background is frequent but does not help in the differentiation between malignancy and benignancy. Multinucleated giant cells of the Langhans' type (fig. 14.7) are seen in chronic granulomatous esophagitis (nonspecific, Crohn's disease, or tuberculosis), but also are present in some instances of esophageal carcinoma. Figure 14.8 illustrates such a finding in a case of squamous cell carcinoma of the esophagus.

Large atypical histiocytes or macrophages (figs. 14.9 and 14.10) occasionally are seen in ulcerative esophagitis. In the early experience with esophageal cytology, they were mistaken for undifferentiated malignant cells.

They are now readily identified as nonepithelial cells of chronic inflammatory processes.

Pernicious Anemia. In untreated pernicious anemia, the cells of all squamous epithelia manifest macrocytosis with macronucleosis, and frequent binucleation (as illustrated in fig. 14.11). As was discussed earlier, this finding is nonspecific and also occurs in other types of anemia.

Irradiation Effect. After mediastinal irradiation, the esophageal cells show typical changes of radiation response (RR). The main changes (figs. 14.12 and 14.13) are: cytoplasmic vacuolation, nuclear enlargement, multinucleation, and, in more advanced stages, pyknosis and even karyorrhexis. These changes are not entirely specific for radiation response and can be seen in other processes, especially chronic inflammation.

Columnar Lined Esophagus. In this rare process, the distal third or two-thirds of the esophagus is lined by a single columnar epithelium of the gastric type. Brushings from such epithelium will reveal only sheets of columnar cells of the gastric type, and no squamous cells.

Squamous Cell Carcinoma of the Esophagus

The vast majority of malignant tumors of the esophagus are invasive squamous cell carcinomas. For practical purposes, one should distinguish two subtypes: the well-differentiated squamous cell carcinoma and the poorly differentiated squamous cell carcinoma.

Well-Differentiated Squamous Cell Carcinoma. As was described in chapter 6, this tumor is characterized by large keratinized eosinophilic cells, intercellular bridging, "epithelial pearls," and spindle or fiber cells. The lack of glandular structure and mucus production (best studied by special stains) also are important histological features. In diagnostic cytologic material, several types of malignant squamous cells have been described and they are all seen in esophageal cytology.

Cytology. Well-differentiated squamous cell carcinomas exfoliate a great number of malignant cells, illustrated in figures 14.14 to 14.33. The two characteristic features of squamous malignant cells are the polygonal or irregular cellular shape and the formation of keratin (manifested by cytoplasmic eosinophilia and ringlike perinuclear deposits). Figures 14.14 to 14.19 illustrate the polygonal shape of the cells. Figures 14.18, 14.19, 14.24 and 14.33 illustrate the cytoplasmic eosinophilia. Another characteristic cell shape seen in squamous cell carcinoma is the so-called tadpole cell, illustrated in figures 14.30 to 14.32. The tadpole cell has a large "head" containing the nucleus or nuclei and a long "tail" of cytoplasm, usually keratinized. The nuclei are usually hyperchromatic and irregular in shape. The perinuclear ringlike deposits of keratin are illustrated in figures 14.20 to 14.22. The cells showing such deposits are usually round and have large nuclei with uneven chromatin.

Spindle or Fiber Cells. The cells, as the name indicates, are elongated and fiberlike with a central nucleus, as illustrated in figure 14.23. They usually are keratinized cells, with dark-staining nuclei, often pyknotic, and angulated or irregularly shaped. These nuclear characteristics help in differentiating them from benign folded squamous cells or smooth muscle fibers.

Bird's-eye Cell. This malignant squamous cell is called "bird's eye" because of its unusual configuration. A small malignant cell is surrounded by a large concentric clear area or vacuole, with thick, well-defined walls. The outer cell also has obviously malignant nuclei. They are illustrated in figures 14.24 to 14.29.

Small Round Eosinophilic Cell. This small cell, usually multinucleated, is seen in the material from large and necrotic tumors. The cytoplasm is thick, homogeneous, and with well-defined round contour, as illustrated in figure 14.33.

Poorly Differentiated Squamous Cell Carcinoma. As was described in chapter 6, this tumor is characterized by dark-staining malignant cells which lack keratin formation, intercellular bridging, or other squamous cell characteristics. It also lacks mucous production or glandular formation. The great majority occur at the lower third of the esophagus.

Cytology. In the cytological material, it is impossible to distinguish them from poorly differentiated adenocarcinomas. However, the tumor frequently has less undifferentiated areas, which exfoliate cells with some characteristics of squamous cell carcinoma. The *undifferentiated malignant cell* of squamous cell carcinomas is usually round or oval, and has a large hyperchromatic nucleus, surrounded by scanty basophilic cytoplasm, as illustrated in figures 14.34 to 14.36. There are abundant isolated cells, or loosely arranged groups or irregular sheets, with nuclear crowding and overlapping. The nuclei frequently have large irregular nucleoli and usually are hyperchromatic.

Adenocarcinoma of the Esophagus

The vast majority of adenocarcinomas of the esophagus are situated in the distal third of the organ and often represent an upward extension of gastric adenocarcinomas. More rarely, they are found entirely within the esophagus and represent truly esophageal tumors. The cytological presentation of these tumors is similar to the usual gastric adenocarcinomas and does not merit special description here.

Nonepithelial Malignant Tumors of the Esophagus

These rare tumors are either malignant lymphomas or leiomyosarcomas. We have experience only with one case of Hodgkin's involvement of the esophagus. The cells obtained were similar to those seen in Hodgkin's disease of the stomach (see chap. 15).

Stomach

Normal Stomach

Histology. The surface epithelium of the stomach is a simple tall columnar epithelium. The supranuclear part of the cells is filled by a special type of mucus. The gastric glands are simple branched tubules that have four types of cells: (*a*) chief or zymogenic cells; (*b*) parietal cells; (*c*) mucous neck cells; and (*d*) argentaffin cells. The accurate identification of such cells in exfoliated material is almost impossible and has no clinical application.

Cytology. The cells of the surface epithelium of the stomach may exfoliate singly or, more frequently, in large sheets. When seen laterally (fig. 14.37) in a well-preserved group, they are tall columnar cells with a small oval nucleus, a supranuclear part filled with mucus (sometimes golden yellow or orange in the Papanicolaou staining), and a small infranuclear amount of basophilic

cytoplasm. Occasionally, one lymphocyte can be seen intraepithelially. When seen from the end (fig. 14.38), the sheets have a honeycomb appearance. The nuclei are quite regular in size and in the oval shape. In the less well-preserved preparations, varying degrees of cellular degeneration will be observed. No attempt at cell diagnosis should be made in such poor specimens because of the danger of confusing degenerative changes with malignancy.

Normally, and especially in gastric washing preparations, a large amount of leukocytes, cellular debris, and squamous cells is present (fig. 14.39), making the screening of such material a very time-consuming task. In the preparations from direct-vision brushing, the background is much clearer and there is little interfering material, facilitating the rapid and easy screening of such slides (fig. 14.40). Occasional pools of lymphocytes are seen in material from normal stomachs, but their presence should raise the suspicion of reactive lymphoreticular hyperplasia or malignant lymphoma (see chap. 15 for detailed description).

Benign Lesions of the Stomach

Chronic Atrophic Gastritis. This process is characterized microscopically by partial or complete atrophy of the gastric glands. The pronounced reduction or absence of the parietal cells is the most striking feature. In advanced cases, there is "intestinalization" of the gastric mucosa; the surface epithelium is more cuboidal, and goblet cells are abundant. Villouslike structures are prominent and Paneth cell metaplasia also is striking. The lamina propria contains increased lymphocytic and plasmocytic infiltrates. In patients with pernicious anemia such changes are extreme and frequently are associated with atypical epithelial changes. The increased incidence of gastric carcinoma in such patients is an indirect indication of the premalignant nature of such changes.

Cytology of Atrophic Gastritis. The cells exfoliated in atrophic gastritis are of two main types: "bland" cells and "active" cells. The "bland" cells (figs. 14.41 to 14.43) are characterized by their large nuclei, with a distinct nuclear membrane but very little stainable chromatin, imparting an empty aspect. Occasionally they have small round nucleoli. Goblet cells can be seen in the large sheets of cells. The "active" cells contain hyperchromatic nuclei, one or more large nucleoli, and other atypical features. They are illustrated with the material of peptic ulcer, where they pose a very important problem in differential diagnosis.

Peptic Ulcer

Atypical glandular regeneration occasionally is seen in the margins of peptic ulcers, and chronic gastritis is almost invariably found in the gastric mucosa near chronic peptic ulcers.

Cytology of Gastric Ulcers. In our experience, the atypical cells seen in material exfoliated from gastric ulcers can be subgrouped into four degrees of atypia. The first is characterized by moderate nuclear enlargement, chromatin clumping, and the presence of one or more small round and regular nucleoli (figs. 14.44 to 14.47). They have been called "active cells." The second degree of atypia is characterized by pronounced anisocytosis and anisonucleosis, some nuclear pleomorphism, and the frequent finding of large irregular nucleoli (figs. 14.48 to 14.52). As in the previous degree of atypia, the cells always exfoliate in groups, with reasonably well-preserved cell boundaries and cohesiveness. Mitoses frequently are seen in the large sheets of cells (fig. 14.47), especially from brushing cytology specimens. Goblet cells frequently are seen, and when their nucleus is atypical or pyknotic (as illustrated in fig. 14.48) they should not be confused with malignant signet-ring cells. Neutrophils frequently are seen as inclusions in the cytoplasm of columnar cells (figs. 14.49, 14.50). The finding of hypochromic nuclei is relatively frequent in washing cytology specimens (fig. 14.51). The third degree of atypia is characterized by advanced dyskaryosis, nuclear pleomorphism, with irregular nuclear-shaped heavy chromatin clumping, and large irregular nucleoli (figs. 14.53, 14.54). The fourth degree of atypia is characterized by isolated atypical cells (figs. 14.55, 14.56).

Granulomatous Gastritis

Chronic gastritis with granuloma formation can be a nonspecific type of inflammatory lesion or part of Crohn's disease with gastric involvement, or it can be due to a specific cause such as tuberculosis of the stomach.

Cytology. In addition to the cells already described in atrophic gastritis, the presence of multinucleated giant cells of the Langhans' type (figs. 14.57 and 14.58) is characteristic of this group of lesions.

Gastric Syphilis

The study of two cases revealed two other cell types in addition to Langhans' cells: fibroblasts and epithelioid cells. Fibroblasts (figs. 14.59 and 14.60) are elongated cells, with a central zone containing the nucleus, and one or two tapering elongated tails. The nucleus is oval, with some irregular chromatin distribution, and contains a large round nucleolus. The nucleus frequently is eccentric and there is no clear cell border, with the cytoplasmic and nuclear membrane apparently merging.

Epithelioid cells (figs. 14.61 and 14.62) have very indistinct cytoplasmic borders. The nuclei usually are oval or cigar-shaped, with a coarse chromatin network (many chromatin granules surrounded by clear areas). The cytoplasm is basophilic, with indistinct borders and many filamentous prolongations (tails), imparting a somewhat bizarre shape to the cells.

Malignant Tumors of the Stomach

Adenocarcinoma. This is the most common type of malignant tumor of the stomach. Histologically, there are several types, varying from well-differentiated to bizarre anaplastic patterns. The degree of connective tissue present and of mucin production also varies considerably. There is no practical advantage in subdividing the cases by their predominant histological pattern. Probably the most important factor to be evaluated is the depth of invasion into the gastric wall. The superficial gastric carcinoma (with mucosal or submucosal level of invasion) has a very favorable prognosis, whereas tumors invading the muscularis propria or deeper into the serosa have a very poor prognosis.

Cytology of Well-Differentiated Adenocarcinomas. These tumors exfoliate large sheets or malignant cells (figs. 14.63 to 14.66). The cells show increased chromatin content, not always uneven, and one or two large nucleoli. The cytoplasm is relatively large, and the nucleus is eccentric, touching the cellular border. In some cells, as seen in figures 14.65 and 14.66, a large mucin-filled vacuole displaces and distorts the nucleus (signet-ring cell in a group). In other cells, the mucin-filled vacuoles either are absent or are very small and multiple. The presence of isolated malignant cells is the rule, but most of the material consists of small or large sheets of malignant cells.

Cytology of Undifferentiated Adenocarcinomas. These more anaplastic tumors exfoliate either large irregular sheets (figs. 14.67 to 14.69), small groups loosely arranged (figs. 14.70 to 14.72), or isolated malignant cells (figs. 14.73 to 14.82).

Figures 14.67 to 14.69 illustrate large groups of malignant cells. Most of the cells retain a columnar pattern. The nuclei are round or oval, with moderate anisonucleosis. Each nucleus has at least one large red nucleolus, occasionally irregular in shape. The cytoplasm is scanty, the cell boundaries are not clear, and there is very dense grouping and crowding. The strikingly abnormal nuclei show marked anisokaryosis, prominent lobulation and indentation. Some cells have no cytoplasm and others have very little, with few vacuoles.

Figures 14.70 to 14.72 show small groups of malignant cells. In figure 14.70, the cells show marked anisokaryosis, some nuclei being particularly large. Each nucleus has one or two large irregular nucleoli. The cytoplasm is scanty in some cells and quite abundant in others and has several mucin-filled vacuoles. There is some tendency to a rosettelike arrangement of the cells in some groups (fig. 14.72); the loose connection between the cells is quite obvious. Abnormal mitoses are seen in most of the material obtained by brushing.

Figures 14.73 to 14.82 show isolated malignant cells. Almost every instance of gastric carcinoma will show some isolated malignant cells. Figures 14.73 to 14.77 illustrate examples of extremely anaplastic malignant cells that are seen in poorly differentiated tumors, and are very easily identified as malignant cells.

The most typical cell of gastric carcinoma is the isolated *signet-ring cell,* examples of which are seen in figures 14.78 to 14.82. All show the characteristic large single vacuole filled with mucin, with well-defined walls, that displaces and distorts the nucleus toward the periphery of the cell. The nuclei of these cells show uneven chromatin content and large irregular nucleoli and are easily recognized as malignant. The identification of signet-ring cells is extremely important; in some gastric tumors, especially of the linitis plastica type, they may be the only malignant cells present.

A variant of the signet-ring cells is the "foamy cytoplasm" type, examples of which are illustrated in figures 14.81 and 14.82. The multiple small, ill-defined vacuoles in the cytoplasm produce the foamy appearance of the cell. They are mucin-filled, and the nucleus is displaced to the periphery of the cell, but it is not distorted by the vacuoles. These cells usually are found in cases with typical signet-ring cells also, but they can be the only cell type present, and identifying them as neoplastic can be very difficult.

Nonepithelial and Metastatic Malignant Tumors of the Stomach

Cytology of malignant lymphomas involving the stomach is discussed in detail in chapter 15. A rarer nonepithelial malignant tumor of the stomach is leiomyosarcoma. We have had the opportunity to study two such tumors by cytology. In one, examined by washing cytology, no malignant cells were recovered. In the other, studied by direct-vision biopsy followed by blind washing cytology, the lavage fluid contained large groups of cells, illustrated in figures 14.83 to 14.86, and recognized as malignant smooth muscle cells. The cells have a spindle shape, with a basophilic thick cytoplasm. The presence of numerous mitoses was highly suggestive of a malignant tumor.

Another case of gastric leiomyosarcoma was seen by us through the courtesy of Drs. Tatsuzo Kasugai, Seibi Kobayashi, and Yuri Yoshii of Nagoya, Japan. The cytological material was collected by direct-vision washing cytology and stained by both Papanicolaou and May-Grunwald-Giemsa methods. In Papanicolaou stained material, illustrated in figures 14.87 to 14.90, most of the cells had an elongated, fiberlike shape, somewhat similar to tadpole cells, although some cells were round and the nucleus had a large irregular nucleolus. In the May-Grunwald-Giemsa stained material (figs. 14.91 to 14.96), the large round cells with large irregular nucleoli were most prominent. This cellular presentation is unique, and is probably characteristic of leiomyosarcoma. Militating against the diagnosis of squamous cell carcinoma in the presence of such cellular presentation is the lack of cytoplasmic eosinophilia of the tadpole-like cells, besides the fact that squamous cell carcinomas of the stomach are extremely rare. Militating against the diagnosis of adenocarcinoma is the presence of such elongated fiberlike cells and the absolute absence of cytoplasmic vacuolization. Obviously, more cases of well-studied leiomyosarcomas are needed before the true cellular presentation of such rare tumors is established.

A case of metastatic malignant melanoma, illustrated

in figures 14.97 and 14.98, exfoliated cells with typical melanin granules in the cytoplasm.

Adenocarcinoma of the stomach frequently metastasizes to the peritoneal cavity. Figures 14.99, 14.100, and 14.101 illustrate malignant cells in ascitic fluid of such cases. The tendency to form rosettes (fig. 14.99) and the presence of signet-ring cells (figs. 14.100 and 14.101) are the rule.

Duodenal Drainage

Histology and Cytology of Normal Epithelia

The technique of duodenal drainage recovers cells arising from the epithelium of the duodenum, pancreatic ducts, and biliary tree. Figure 14.102 shows a sheet of duodenal epithelium, with the cells seen from the end; the honeycomb pattern is typical. Figure 14.103 shows a lateral view of the columnar cells of the duodenum, with their striated border. The primary pancreatic ducts' epithelium is lined by a low columnar epithelium with occasional goblet cells. Figure 14.104 demonstrates a sheet of exfoliated ductal cells with their dark-staining oval nuclei. The cells are polygonal in shape and have a relatively small amount of cytoplasm. A lateral view of the cells is seen in figure 14.105.

The columnar cells of the biliary tree are taller than their counterparts in the pancreas, but they cannot be distinguished with certainty from the pancreatic ductal cell in the exfoliative cytology material.

The background of the smears prepared from duodenal drainage always is composed of large amounts of degenerated cells of unindentifiable origin. In our experience, it is not possible to identify liver cells as such, as some authors have claimed to do.

The diagnosis of inflammatory processes in the pancreaticobiliary tree or in the duodenal mucosa also is not possible by exfoliative cytology.

Cytology of Malignant Lesions

Malignant cells from the tumors arising in the duodenum, pancreas, or biliary tract, when present, are identified easily because of their large size and anaplastic features, in comparison with the normal columnar cells. Unfortunately, the duodenal contents are subject to rapid degeneration, and this is a major obstacle in accurate identification of the cells.

Figures 14.106 to 14.111 illustrate groups of malignant cells obtained by duodenal drainage. Figures 14.106 and 14.107 are from cases of adenocarcinoma of the duodenum. The cells have large irregular cytoplasmic vacuoles and hyperchromatic nuclei with prominent nucleoli.

Figures 14.108 to 14.110 illustrate cells from cases of adenocarcinoma of the pancreas. They show the same general characteristics as adenocarcinoma cells of the digestive tract, and their origin from the pancreas cannot be ascertained by cytologic criteria.

Figure 14.111 is from a patient with adenocarcinoma of the gall bladder. The pattern shows a greater tendency to isolated cells, but this criterion is not specific enough to identify their origin in a particular case.

Microscopic Identification of Biliary Crystals

Biliary cholesterol crystals are readily identified in wet preparations by their characteristic platelike, notched-corner appearance (figs. 14.112 to 14.114). Calcium bilirubinate conglomerates are golden yellow or brown orange granules that always accompany the cholesterol crystals, but they can occur alone.

Parasites

The morphology of parasites and their eggs that can be identified in duodenal contents is the object of many excellent texts. Of special interest, because of its presence in relatively good preservation in Papanicolaou stained slides, is *Giardia lamblia* (figs. 14.115 to 14.118). In fresh wet preparations they are recognized by their cup-like shape and their motility.

In one case, larvae of *Strongyloides stercoralis* were identified in the fresh wet preparation. The fixed material did not allow identification of the larvae because of their poor fixation and staining.

Colon

Histology and Cytology of Normal Colonic Epithelium

The surface epithelium of the colonic mucosa is composed of tall columnar cells, with intervening goblet cells in large numbers, as illustrated by figure 14.119. Exfoliated cells also are tall columnar cells (fig. 14.120).

Benign Lesions

Chronic Ulcerative Colitis and "Granulomatous Colitis." In these inflammatory bowel diseases, the surface epithelium of the colon may show striking changes. In chronic ulcerative colitis, there is an increased incidence of carcinoma of the colon, and the finding of highly atypical changes, of the type illustrated in figures 14.121 to 14.123, has been interpreted as a premalignant change or carcinoma in situ. Figure 14.121 illustrates, in low power, the atypical glands with irregular branching and cellular crowding in the surface epithelium. Figures 14.122 and 14.123 illustrate the glandular and cellular atypia (dark-staining nuclei with marked anisonucleosis) of carcinoma in situ. Exfoliative cytology material in chronic ulcerative colitis is characterized by several types of atypical cells. Figures 14.124 and 14.125 illustrate the "bland" cells; these are large cells with marked nuclear enlargement. Figures 14.126 to 14.128 illustrate "active" cells; these are characterized by a large nucleus with increased chromatin content, unevenly distributed, and by one or two red nucleoli.

Figures 14.129 to 14.132 illustrate a more advanced degree of cellular atypia seen in chronic ulcerative colitis. These cells are characterized by nuclear polymorphism, unclear cellular borders, and crowding. These cells can easily be confused with malignant cells. At this stage of our knowledge, we cannot state with certainty whether they are shed by microscopic foci of carcinoma in situ or from areas of atypical epithelial hyperplasia.

Figures 14.133 to 14.136 illustrate nonepithelial cells seen in the presence of chronic ulcerative colitis and granulomatous colitis. Figure 14.133 shows a multinucleated giant cell, with a ground-class cytoplasm and several cigar-shaped nuclei. Figures 14.134 and 14.135 show large immature-looking lymphoid cells. Their presence should not lead to a diagnosis of malignant lymphoma of the colon.

Figure 14.136 shows an extremely large naked nucleus, probably nonepithelial in nature. Similar nuclei are found in very active stages of long-standing ulcerative colitis.

Irradiation Proctitis. Cytology of this lesion is characterized by nuclear enlargement, some increase in chromatin content, and moderate anisonucleosis, as illustrated in figure 14.137.

Malignant Lesions of the Colon

Adenocarcinoma of the Colon. This tumor is characterized by large irregular cells, of adenocarcinoma type,

as shown in figures 14.138 to 14.155. The nuclei are pleomorphic and frequently have a prominent red nucleolus. In the well-preserved material the diagnosis is easily made, but in degenerated material or in the presence of excessive fecal material, the diagnosis is very difficult.

The prominent red nucleoli are well illustrated in figures 14.138 to 14.145. The anaplastic, irregularly shaped nuclei are best seen in figures 14.146 and 14.147. Extremely large nuclei are illustrated in figures 14.145 to 14.152. The presence of large and multilobulated nuclei is seen in figures 14.150 to 14.152. The presence of signet-ring cells or more typically of large vacuoles in malignant cells is frequent, and is illustrated in figures 14.153 to 14.155

II. MORPHOLOGY OF CELLS STAINED BY OTHER METHODS: ACRIDINE ORANGE, SHORR'S POLYCHROMIC, AND MAY-GRUNWALD-GIEMSA

Acridine-Orange Fluorescence Microscopy Method

The use of Acridine Orange permits a combination of morphological and biochemical study of the exfoliated cells. Acridine Orange combines with the nuclei acids of the cell, and under ultraviolet excitation DNA fluoresces yellowish green and RNA fluoresces red. According to the pH of the buffer solution, the amount of either cytoplasmic/nucleolar or nuclear fluorescence is increased. We employed the technique of Bertalanffy, which applies a pH of 6, emphasizing the red fluorescence of RNA. However, the DNA fluorescence is still very evident, and the overall picture gives as much cellular morphology as the Papanicolaou stained cells. The Acridine-Orange method is particularly helpful in slides heavily contaminated with blood, because the red cells do not fluoresce.

Figures 14.156 to 14.158 show normal columnar gastric cells. The oval nuclei with their small, evenly distributed chromatin granules are easily seen by their yellowish green fluorescence, and the cytoplasm is shown by its faint red fluorescence.

Figures 14.159 to 14.161 show gastric columnar cells from patients with gastric ulcer. The nuclear enlargement is prominent, and the nuclei have coarse chromatin granules. The strong cytoplasmic red fluorescence is striking, and should not lead to a false-positive diagnosis. The morphological study of the entire group of cells permits the conclusion that they are atypical yet benign cells.

Figures 14.162 and 14.163 show malignant squamous cells. The large polygonal cell has a very strong red cytoplasmic fluorescence that partially obscures the green nuclei and their red nucleoli. Figure 14.163 shows a malignant pearl.

Figures 14.164 to 14.172 illustrate cases of adenocarcinoma of the stomach. It is clear that morphological detail can be seen easily. The background is completely black, making the screening extremely easy, even in the presence of blood.

Figures 14.168 to 14.172, taken under $\times$ 1,250 magnification, show how the nuclear morphological detail is clearly seen.

Shorr's Polychromic Staining Method

This staining method gives excellent cytoplasmic staining, facilitating the study of characteristics such as cell shapes, cytoplasmic vacuoles, and degree of keratinization of squamous cells. However, the nuclear stain, Biebrich Scarlet, is less adequate than usual nuclear stains such as hematoxylin. Adequate fixation and optimal cell preservation are extremely important for good nuclear staining; but even under such optimal conditions not all cells will show adequate nuclear staining. This is especially true for large sheets of cells, where the cells in the core will show minimal staining, sometimes only a few chromocenters being stained. We have found that adding 0.1% (final concentration) DMSO to the fixative produces better nuclear staining.

Figure 14.173 shows examples of atypical columnar cells, with prominent red nucleoli and enlarged nuclei, from a case of gastric benign ulcer. Figures 14.174 and 14.175 are from cases of gastric adenocarcinoma. The signet-ring cell seen in figure 14.68 is another example of good staining by this technique.

May-Grunwald-Giemsa Staining Method

This method is especially useful when a malignant lymphoma is suspected, because the nonepithelial cells are recognized easily by their familial hematological morphology. Figures 14.176 to 14.180 were provided by Dr. Tatsuzo Kasugai and his associates from the Department of Internal Medicine, Aichi Cancer Center Hospital, Nagoya, Japan, and illustrate cells from cases of gastric carcinoma.

Figures 14.176 and 14.177 show groups of cells in a palisade arrangement, suggesting their glandular origin. Figures 14.178 to 14.180 illustrate loosely arranged cells, with large nuclei characterized by a very irregular chromatin pattern, each one having large irregular nucleoli. Some of the cells have cytoplasmic vacuoles.

Several figures in chapter 15 illustrate the use of MGG stain in cases of malignant lymphoma.

15

Cytology of Malignant Lymphomas and Reactive Lymphoreticular Hyperplasia of the Gastrointestinal Tract

Our experience with malignant lymphomas of the stomach has indicated that, in addition to an increased number of lymphocytes (fig. 15.1), three main types of malignant cells are demonstrable, as Rubin and Massey (242) have previously shown:

Lymphoid Cell (Undifferentiated Lymphocyte). A round cell, with a diameter two or more times that of a normal lymphocyte; with a small rim or ground-glass cytoplasm, and with a round nucleus with a large, usually single, nucleolus and a distinct nuclear membrane (fig. 15.2 to 15.5).

Reticulum Cell. A usually round, occasionally irregular cell, with a moderate amount of ground-glass cytoplasm. The nucleus usually is indented with one or more nucleoli. The nuclear membrane is thin and the chromatin content is delicate (figs. 15.6 to 15.14).

Sternberg-Reed Cell. A large binucleated (occasionally multinucleated) cell, with fairly abundant cytoplasm. The nuclei are "mirror images" with irregular chromatin content and one nucleolus per nucleus or nuclear lobe (figs. 15.15 and 15.16).

The differentiation between the "lymphoid" and "reticulum" or "histiocytic" cells and small anaplastic adenocarcinoma cells is presented in table 15.1.

The most helpful criteria in this differentiation are those of Rubin and Massey (242), Shida, Koike, and Kotaka (259), Shida and Tsuda (260), and our own observations (208):

a) The malignant lymphomas never form cohesive groups or clumps; an isolated cell pattern is the absolute rule. However, these isolated cells can be seen in loosely arranged clusters, as is illustrated in figures 15.17 and 15.18. In this particular patient, the final histological diagnosis was Hodgkin's disease of the stomach. In the May-Grunwald-Giemsa material, only isolated cells of the reticular type were seen, many of them with mitotic figures (figures 15.19 to 15.21). Occasionally adenocarcinomas will present an isolated cell pattern, but the usual distribution is the grouping into cohesive aggregates and clusters (the more typical being palisades and rosette).

b) The chromatin pattern is the next most useful criterion. Nonepithelial cells usually have a regular pattern of small chromatin masses surrounded by clear spaces, and the epithelial cells usually have an irregular

TABLE 15.1

DIFFERENTIATION BETWEEN MALIGNANT LYMPHOMA CELLS AND UNDIFFERENTIATED ADENOCARCINOMA CELLS

	Reticulum Cell	Lymphoid Cell	Adenocarcinoma Cell
Nuclear changes			
Chromatin	Regular delicate pattern: closely packed in small masses surrounded by clear spaces	Regular pattern: closely packed in small masses surrounded by clear spaces; occasionally coarse	Irregular pattern: condensation in large masses, leaving large empty spaces
Nucleoli	Large, irregular in shape, and frequently multiple	Usually a large single round one; sometimes absent	Usually multiple, large, irregular in shape and size
Nuclear membrane	Usually thin and delicate	Usually thick	Usually thick
Nuclear shape	Round or oval, frequently indented or budding	Usually round or oval; occasionally angulated	Usually oval or round
Multinucleation	Sternberg-Reed type	Rare	Frequent, associated with anisonucleosis
Cytoplasmic changes			
Amount and distribution	Scanty; perinuclear ring	Very scanty; perinuclear rim	Variable; eccentric nuclei
Cell membrane	Usually not clear	Clear	Usually not clear
Vacuolization	Small vacuoles rarely seen	Usually absent	Large irregular vacuoles usually seen
Phagocytosis	Occasionally seen	Rare	Occasionally seen
Interrelationships of cells			
Grouping	Isolated scattered cell pattern; never form cohesive groups	Isolated scattered cell pattern; never form cohesive groups	Usually form cohesive groups or clusters; very rarely only isolated cells
Anisokaryosis	Moderate	Rare	Frequent
Anisocytosis	Moderate	Rare	Frequent
Engulfment of one cell by another	Occasionally seen	Usually absent	Frequent

SOURCE: Prolla, Kobayashi, and Kirsner (208).
NOTE: Papanicolaou stain.

pattern of large chromatin masses and large, empty nuclear spaces.

c) A less reliable but useful criterion is cytoplasmic vacuolization. The nonepithelial cells usually have no vacuoles or only faintly visible ones; the epithelial cell, on the other hand, usually has large vacuoles (the most typical being the signet-ring cell type).

Other features are much less reliable and only a combination of several can be accepted for diagnosis. However, the three criteria mentioned above usually are found if the smears are of good technical quality.

No complete correlation was found between these cell types and the histological diagnoses, except in a few lymphomas of the lymphocytic types that showed only lymphocytes and "lymphoid" malignant cells. However, in the less differentiated lymphocytic lymphomas the malignant cells were indistinguishable from the "reticulum cells." In some cases of histiocytic lymphomas, Reed-Sternberg cells were noted. This lack of correlation is understandable, since the histological classification is based upon the predominant cell type only. With very few exceptions, the tumor always manifests some mixed cellularity; this is typically exemplified by the malignant lymphoma of mixed cell type where there is neoplastic proliferation of histiocytes and lymphocytes, without appreciable predominance of either cell type. Diagnostic cytology by gastric washing and Papanicolaou staining can facilitate a positive diagnosis of malignant lymphoma in a fairly high number of cases (64% in our series) but cannot distinguish between the histological types of lymphoma. Rubin and Massey (242), in their analysis of the first cases of this series, had mentioned this problem and also quoted the work of Moore and Reagan (186), showing a similar problem in the analysis of the cellular material obtained by lymph-node imprint from various types of lymphomas.

In more than 3,000 cytological examinations of the stomach performed during the same period, in patients with benign conditions or adenocarcinomas, two errors were made that have some relationship to the lymphoma problem:

a) In one instance of adenocarcinoma, the malignant cells were uniformly rather small, isolated (never forming groups), and with scanty cytoplasm, leading to an incorrect diagnosis of malignant lymphoma rather than carcinoma.

b) In another patient, a large number of pools of lymphocytes were seen; some appearing immature and suggesting a false diagnosis of malignant lymphoma. The final diagnosis was reactive lymphoreticular hyperplasia or pseudolymphoma of the stomach.

After this experience, two other instances of pseudolymphoma (figs. 15.22 and 15.23) were studied by exfoliative cytology, and the presence of plasma cells mixed with the lymphocytes facilitated correct interpretation of the cellular material as benign in origin (147, 208). However, and especially in material stained with May-Grunwald-Giemsa staining method, plasma cells also can be seen in cases of malignant lymphoma. Figures 15.24 to 15.26 illustrate several plasma cells seen in a patient with histiocytic lymphoma of the stomach, from the collection of Dr. Kasugai and his associates from Nagoya, Japan. It is interesting that the two cases of pseudolymphoma of the series of Klayman et al. (139), originally thought to be malignant lymphomas, were reported as negative for malignant cells.

As was seen in the previous chapter, a somewhat similar problem was found in the colon; in two cases of chronic ulcerative colitis, very immature-looking lymphoid cells were recovered. However, because of the rarity of true lymphoma of the colon and the association of inflammatory bowel diseases such as ulcerative and granulomatous colitis with heavy lymphocytic infiltrates, no positive report was issued. Also, the previously mentioned experience of Galambos (79, 81) in our laboratory helped to establish the diagnosis.

Illustrations

81

Fig. 3.1. (*a*) Distal part of the gastrofiberscope, showing the brush for cytology extending through the bent instrument. (*b*) Distal end of the esophagofiberscope, showing the biopsy forceps protruding through the bent instrument.

Fig. 3.2. Technique of smearing the brush on the microscope glass slide: quick circular movement while applying moderate pressure of the brush against the glass slide.

Fig. 3.3. Immediate fixation in 95° ethyl alcohol, before any drying occurs, is extremely important when using Papanicolaou's staining method.

Figs. 12.1 and 12.2. Groups of malignant cells from a case of adenocarcinoma of the sigmoid colon, obtained by brushing under direct vision through a fiber-colonoscope (Papanicolaou staining). × 1,000.

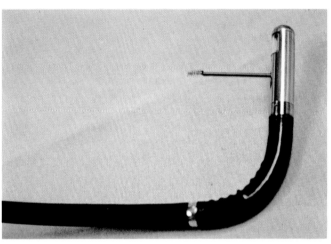

3.1*a*

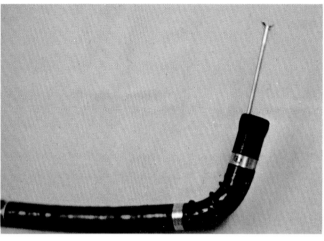

3.1*b*

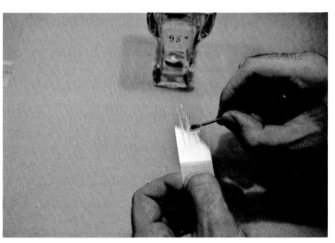

3.2

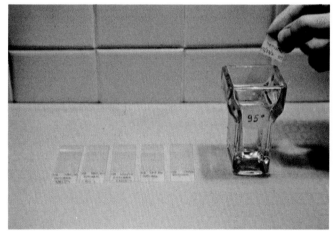

3.3

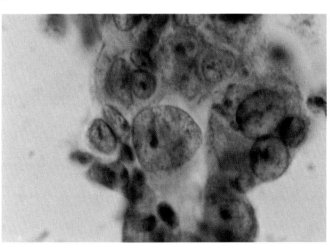

12.1

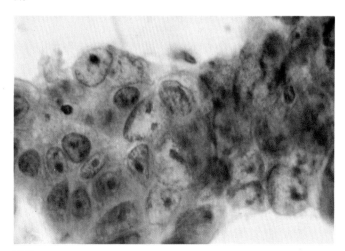

12.2

82

Figs. 14.1 and 14.2. Normal esophagus; superficial squamous cells (Papanicolaou stain). × 400.

Fig. 14.3. Normal esophagus; superficial squamous cells (Pap stain). × 1,000.

Fig. 14.4. Normal esophagus; benign "pearl" formation (Pap stain). × 400.

Fig. 14.5. Normal esophagus; intermediate layer cells (Pap stain). × 1,000.

Fig. 14.6. Chronic esophagitis; basal layer cells (Pap stain). × 1,000.

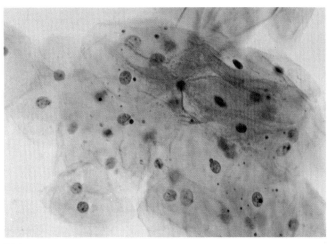

14.1

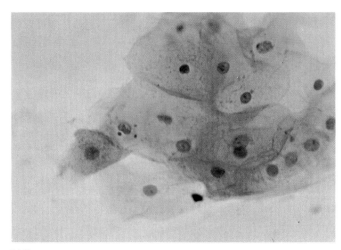

14.2

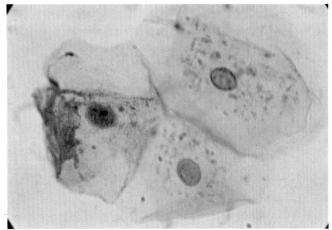

14.3

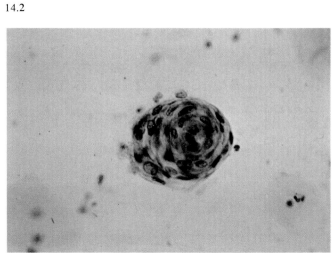

14.4

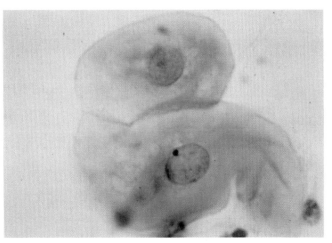

14.5

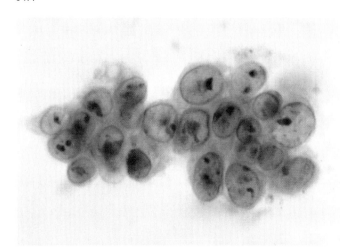

14.6

83

Fig. 14.7. Chronic granulomatous esophagitis; multinucleated giant cell (Pap stain). × 400.

Fig. 14.8. Squamous cell carcinoma of the esophagus; multinucleated giant cell (Pap stain). × 1,000.

Figs. 14.9 and 14.10. Chronic esophagitis and achalasia; tissue macrophages (Pap stain). × 1,000.

Fig. 14.11. Pernicious anemia; binucleated squamous cell (Pap stain). × 400.

Fig. 14.12. Irradiation effect on squamous cells; the patient had mediastinal lymphoma and received 6,000 rads to this area (Pap stain). × 1,000.

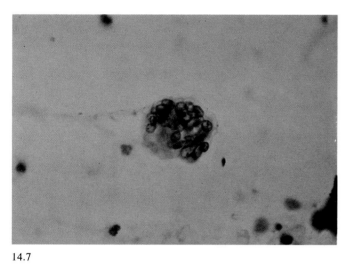

14.7

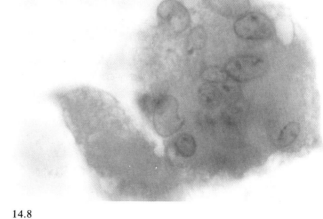

14.8

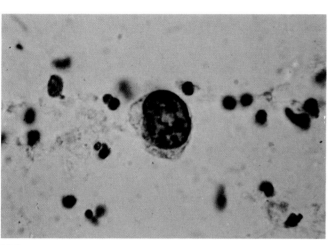

14.9

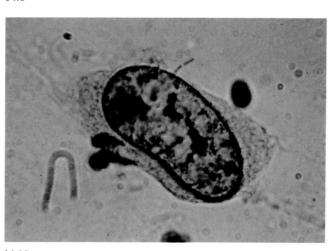

14.10

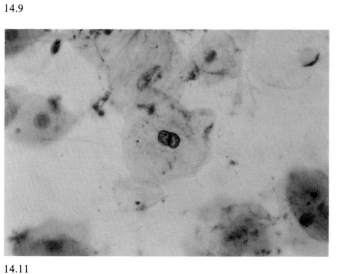

14.11

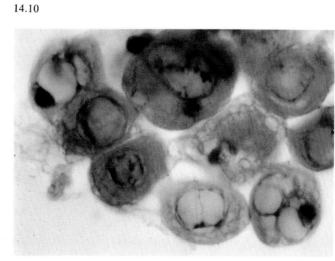

14.12

84

Fig. 14.13. Irradiation effect on squamous cells; the patient had mediastinal lymphoma and received 6,000 rads to this area (Pap stain). × 1,000.

Figs. 14.14 to 14.18. Squamous cell carcinoma of the esophagus; polygonal cells with varying degrees of keratinization (Pap stain). × 400 (figs. 14.14 and 14.17) and × 1,000 (figs. 14.15, 14.16, 14.18).

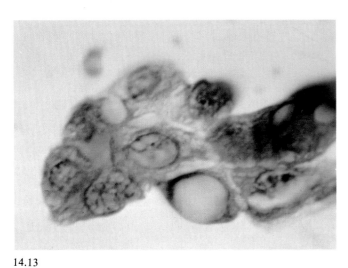

14.13

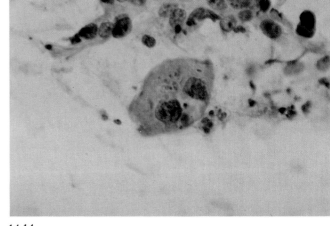

14.14

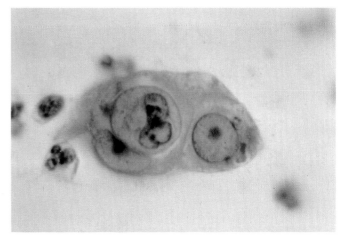

14.15

14.16

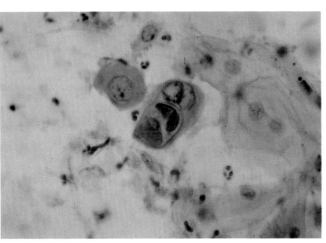

14.17

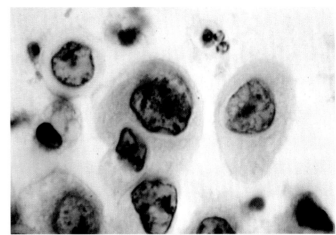

14.18

85

Fig. 14.19. Squamous cell carcinoma of the esophagus; polygonal cells with varying degrees of keratinization (Pap stain). × 1,000.

Figs. 14.20 to 14.22. Squamous cell carcinoma of the esophagus; round cell with perinuclear ringlike keratin deposits (Pap stain). × 1,000.

Fig. 14.23. Squamous cell carcinoma of the esophagus; typical fiber cells (Pap stain). × 400.

Fig. 14.24. Squamous cell carcinoma of the esophagus; typical bird's-eye cells (Pap stain). × 400.

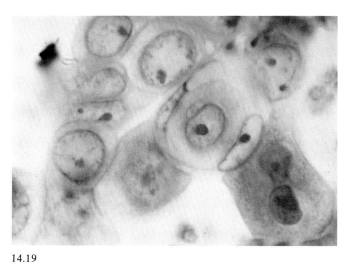

14.19

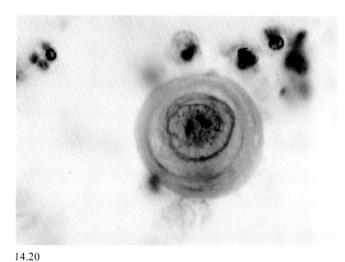

14.20

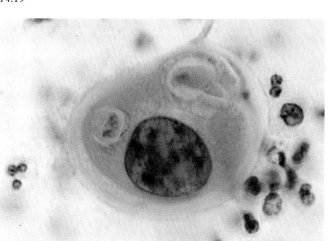

14.21

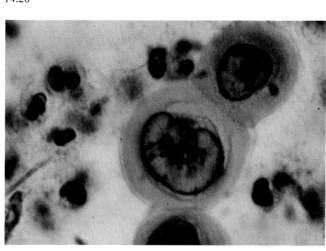

14.22

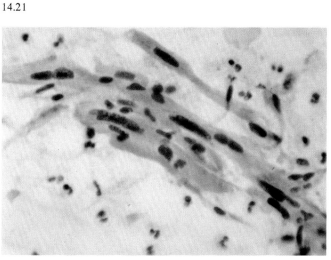

14.23

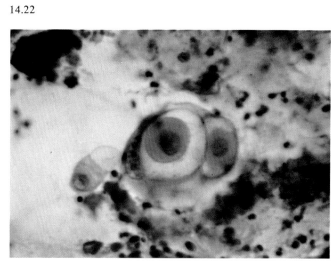

14.24

Figs. 14.25 to 14.29. Squamous cell carcinoma of the esophagus; typical bird's-eye cells (Pap stain). × 400 (figs. 14.25 and 14.26) and × 1,000 (figs. 14.27 to 14.29).

Fig. 14.30. Squamous cell carcinoma of the esophagus; tadpole cells (Pap stain). × 1,000.

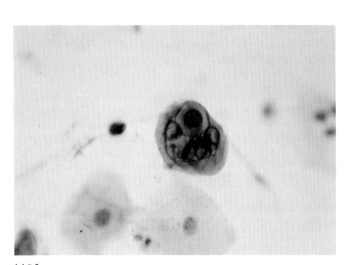

14.25

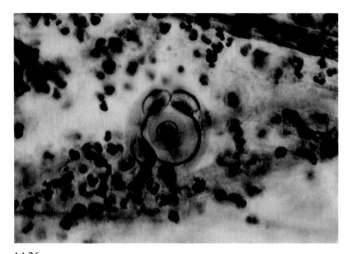

14.26

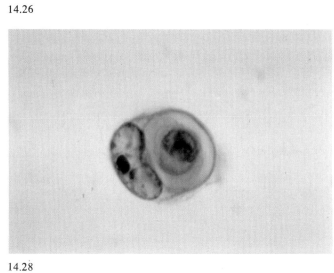

14.28

14.27

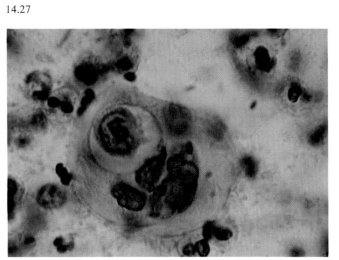

14.29

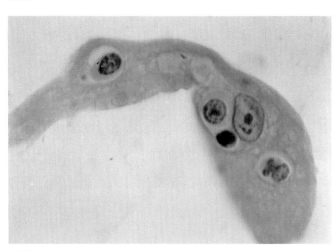

14.30

Figs. 14.31 and 14.32. Squamous cell carcinoma of the esophagus; tadpole cells (Pap stain). × 1,000 (fig. 14.31) and × 400 (fig. 14.32).

Fig. 14.33. Squamous cell carcinoma of the esophagus; round eosinophilic cell (Pap stain). × 1,000.

Figs. 14.34 to 14.36. Undifferentiated carcinoma of the esophagus; undifferentiated malignant cells (Pap stain). × 1,000.

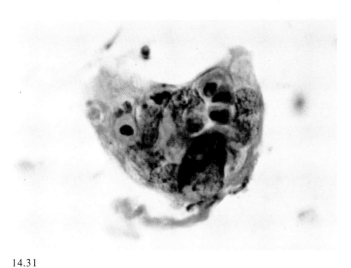

14.31

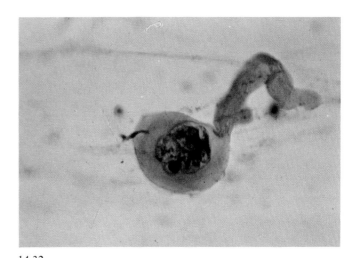

14.32

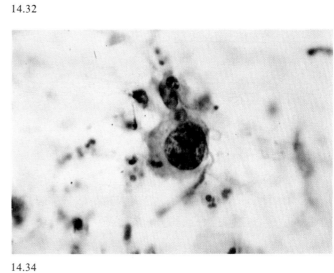

14.33

14.34

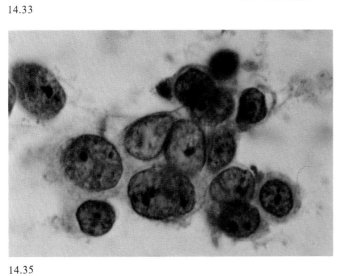

14.35

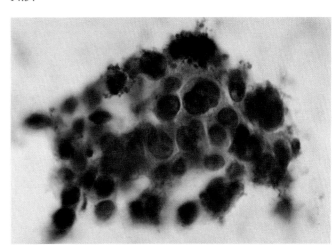

14.36

Fig. 14.37. Normal stomach; columnar cells seen laterally (Pap stain). × 1,000.

Fig. 14.38. Normal stomach; columnar cells seen from the end (Pap stain). × 400.

Fig. 14.39. Adenocarcinoma of the cardia; group of malignant cells against a heavy background of squamous cells and leukocytes, in washing cytology preparation (Pap stain). × 400.

Fig. 14.40. Adenocarcinoma of the stomach; group of malignant cells against a clear background, in a brushing cytology preparation (Pap stain). × 400.

Figs. 14.41 and 14.42. Chronic gastritis; typical groups of "bland" cells (Pap stain). × 1,000.

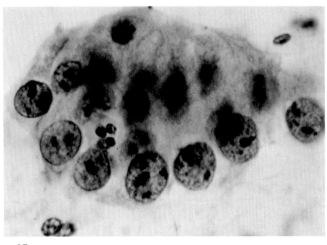

14.37

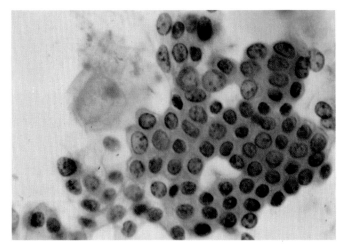

14.38

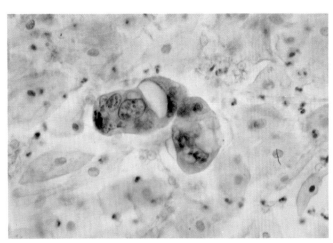

14.39

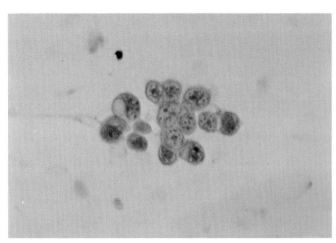

14.40

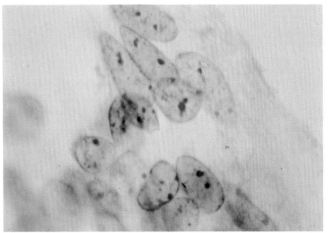

14.41

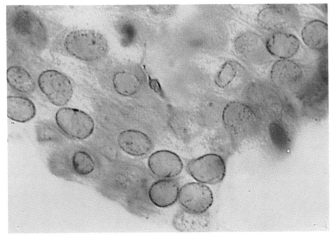

14.42

89

Fig. 14.43. Chronic gastritis; typical groups of "bland" cells (Pap stain). × 1,000.

Figs. 14.44 to 14.47. Benign gastric ulcer; sheets of "active" cells (Pap stain). × 1,000.

Fig. 14.48. Benign gastric ulcer; groups of atypical cells of moderate degree of atypia (Pap stain). × 1,000.

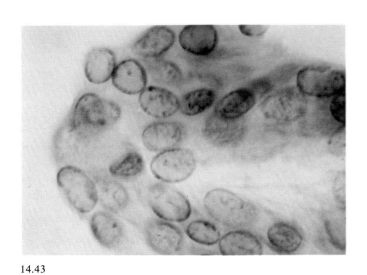

14.43

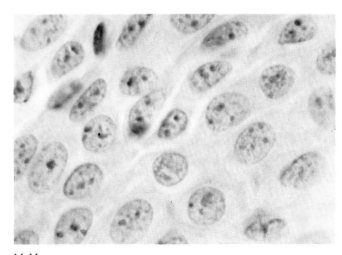

14.44

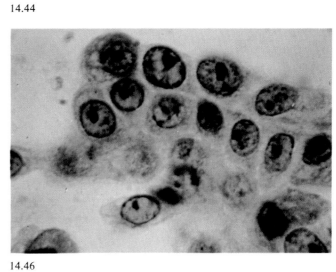

14.45

14.46

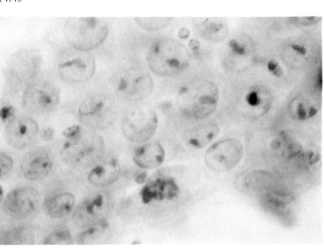

14.47

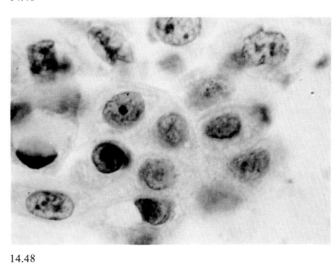

14.48

Fig. 14.49 to 14.52. Benign gastric ulcer; groups of atypical cells of moderate degree of atypia (Pap stain). × 1,000.

Figs. 14.53 and 14.54. Benign gastric ulcer; groups of atypical cells with advanced degree of atypia (Pap stain). × 1,000.

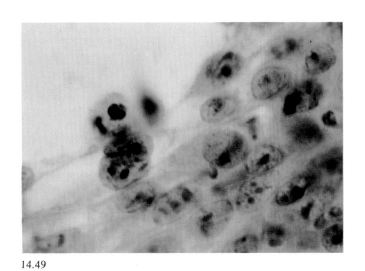

14.49

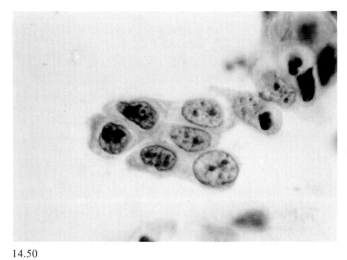

14.50

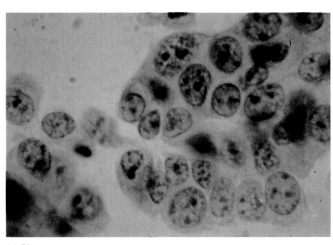

14.52

14.51

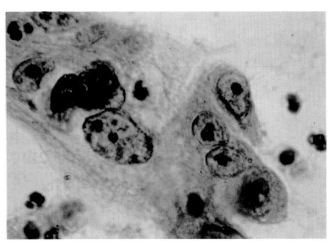

14.53

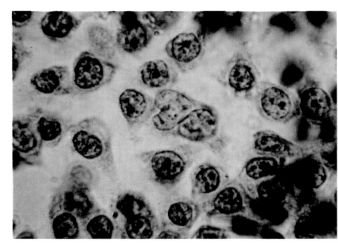

14.54

91

Figs. 14.55 and 14.56. Benign gastric ulcer; isolated atypical cells, difficult to differentiate from malignant cells (Pap stain). × 1,000.

Figs. 14.57 and 14.58. Chronic granulomatous gastritis; multinucleated giant cells (Pap stain). × 1,000.

Figs. 14.59 and 14.60. Gastric syphilis; groups of epithelioid cells and fibroblasts (Pap stain). × 400.

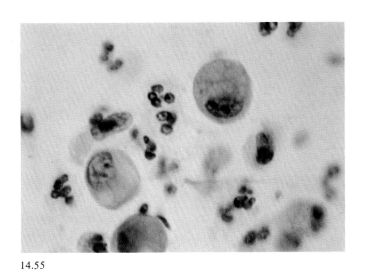

14.55

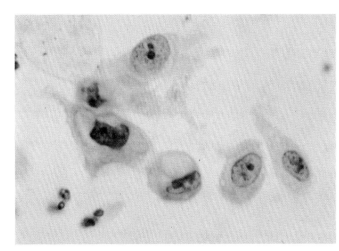

14.56

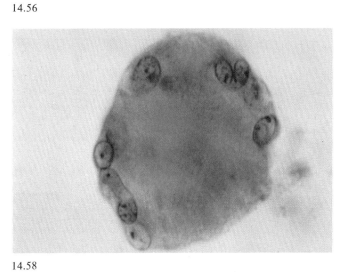

14.57

14.58

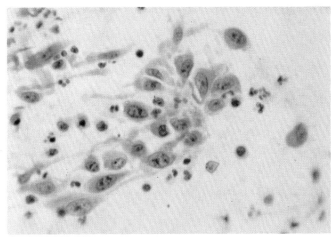

14.59

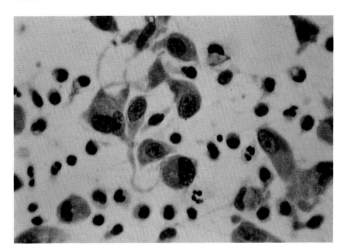

14.60

92

Figs. 14.61 and 14.62. Gastric syphilis; groups of epithelioid cells and fibroblasts (Pap stain) × 400.

Figs. 14.63 to 14.66. Adenocarcinoma of the stomach; well-differentiated adenocarcinoma cells in small groups (Pap stain). × 1,000 (figs. 14.63, 14.64) and × 400 (figs. 14.65, 14.66).

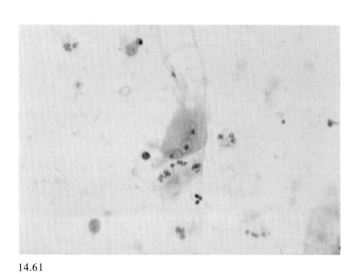

14.61

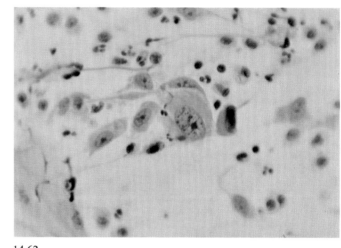

14.62

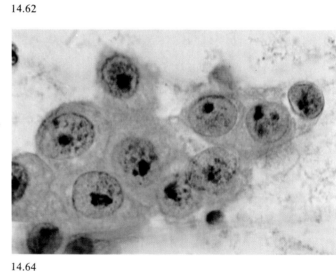

14.63

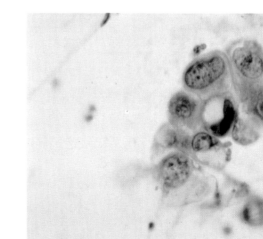

14.64

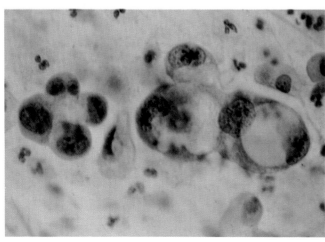

14.65

14.66

Figs. 14.67 to 14.69. Adeno-carcinoma of the stomach; groups of relatively undif-ferentiated malignant cells (Pap stain). × 400.

Figs. 14.70 to 14.72. Adeno-carcinoma of the stomach; small groups of anaplastic adenocarcinoma cells (Pap stain). × 1,000 (figs. 14.70, 14.72) and × 400 (fig. 14.71).

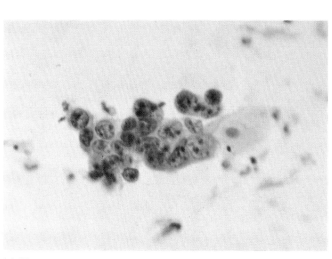

14.67

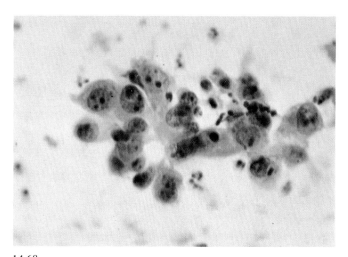

14.68

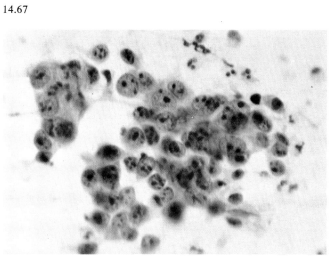

14.69

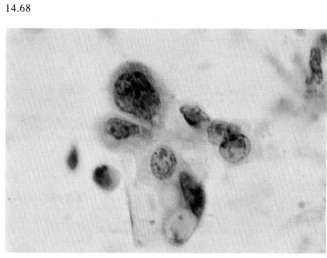

14.70

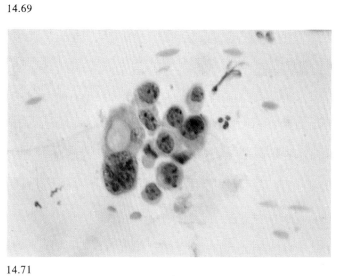

14.71

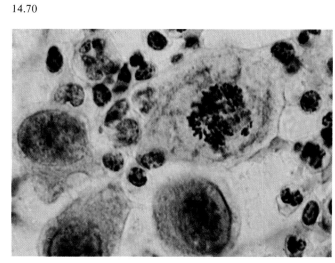

14.72

Figs. 14.73 to 14.77. Adenocarcinoma of the stomach;
isolated anaplastic malignant cells (Pap stain).
× 1,000.

Fig. 14.78. Adenocarcinoma
of the stomach; typical signet-
ring cells (Shorr stain).
× 1,000.

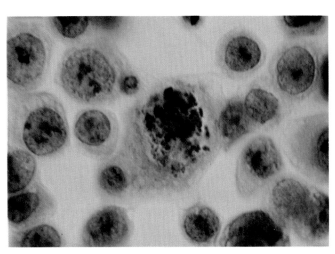

14.73

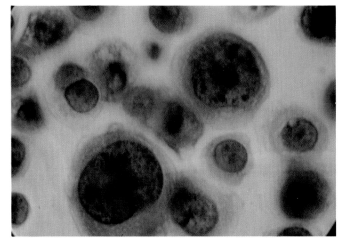

14.74

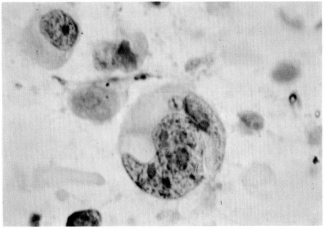

14.75

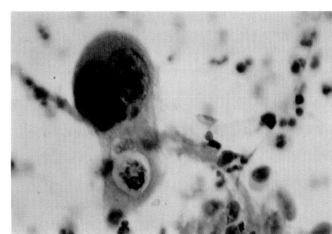

14.76

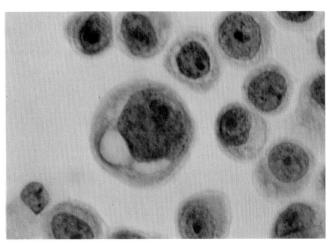

14.77

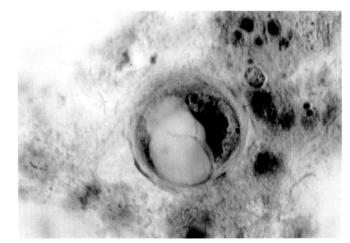

14.78

95

Figs. 14.79 and 14.80. Adeno-carcinoma of the stomach; typical signet-ring cells (Pap stain). × 1,000.

Figs. 14.81 and 14.82. Adeno-carcinoma of the stomach; isolated malignant cells with "foamy" cytoplasm (Pap stain). × 1,000.

Figs. 14.83 and 14.84. Leio-myosarcoma of the stomach; large groups of spindle-shaped cells, many of which are in mitosis (Pap stain). × 1,000.

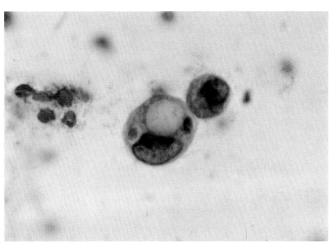

14.79

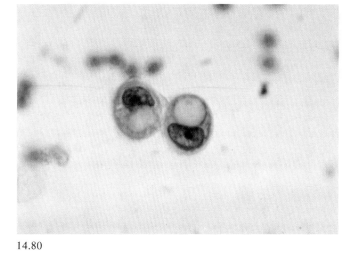

14.80

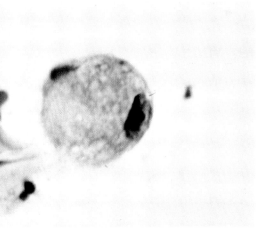

14.81

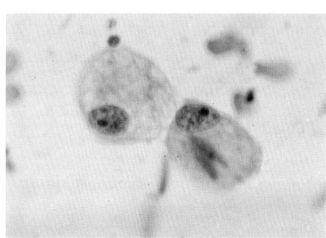

14.82

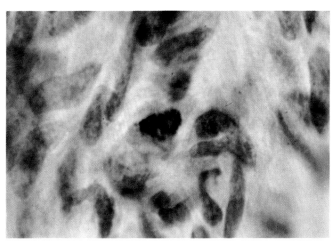

14.83

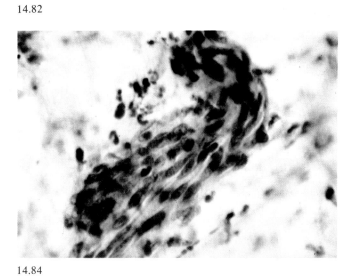

14.84

Figs. 14.85 and 14.86. Leio-myosarcoma of the stomach; large groups of spindle-shaped cells, many of which are in mitosis (Pap stain). $\times$ 1,000 (fig. 14.83) and $\times$ 400 (fig. 14.84).

Figs. 14.87 to 14.90. Leio-myosarcoma of the stomach; isolated malignant cells, many of which have a spindle shape (Pap stain). $\times$ 1,000. (Case studied by us by courtesy of Drs. Kasugai, Kobayashi, and Yoshii, from Nagoya, Japan.)

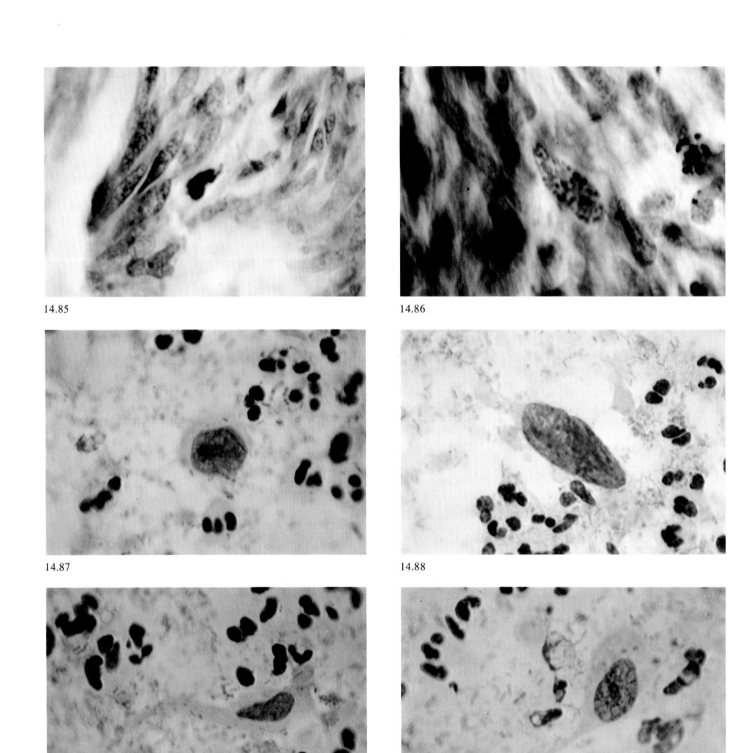

14.85

14.86

14.87

14.88

14.89

14.90

Figs. 14.91 to 14.96. Leio-
myosarcoma of the stomach;
groups of malignant cells,
of undifferentiated nature,
some of them with a spindle
shape. Same case as figs.
14.87 to 14.90 (May-
Grunwald-Giemsa stain).
× 1,000.

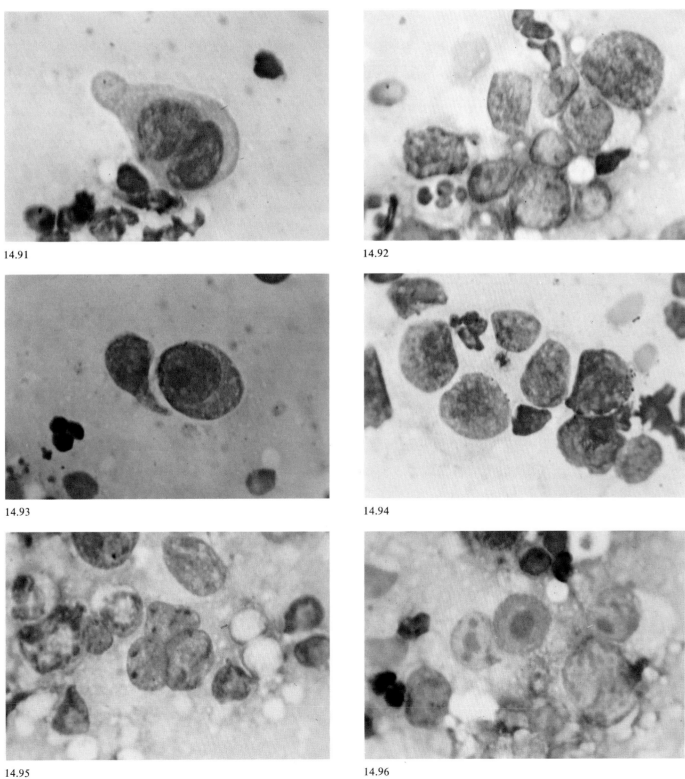

14.91

14.92

14.93

14.94

14.95

14.96

98

Figs. 14.97 and 14.98. Metastatic malignant melanoma of the stomach; groups of cells with brown pigment granules in the cytoplasm (Pap stain). × 400.

Figs. 14.99 to 14.101. Ascitic fluid in metastatic adenocarcinoma of the stomach; typical rosette formation (fig. 14.99), and signet-ring cells (figs. 14.100, 14.101) (Pap stain). × 1,000 (except fig. 14.99, which is × 400).

Fig. 14.102. Normal duodenal drainage; sheets of duodenal cells seen from the end (Pap stain). × 400.

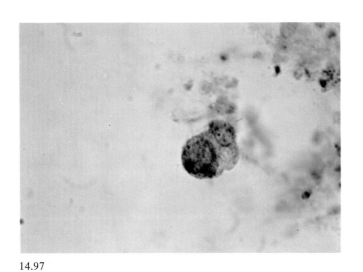

14.97

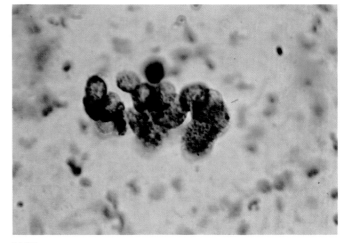

14.98

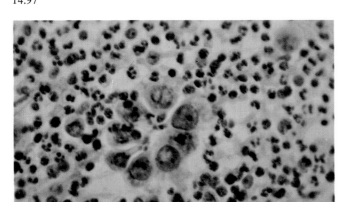

14.99

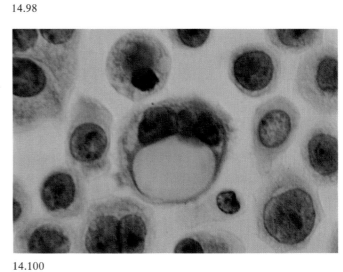

14.100

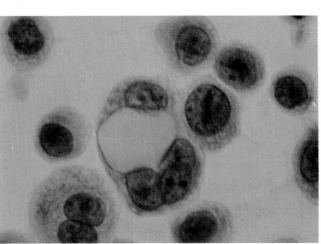

14.101

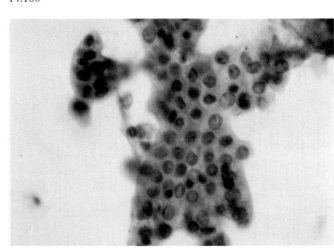

14.102

99

Fig. 14.103. Normal duodenal drainage; duodenal cells with typical brush borders (Pap stain). × 1,000.

Figs. 14.104 and 14.105. Normal duodenal drainage; probable ductal cells (Pap stain). × 400.

Figs. 14.106 and 14.107. Primary adenocarcinoma of the duodenum; groups of malignant cells (Pap stain). × 1,000.

Fig. 14.108. Adenocarcinoma of the pancreas; small groups of malignant cells (Pap stain). × 1,000.

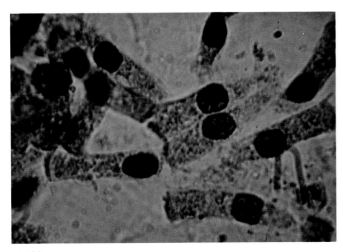

14.103

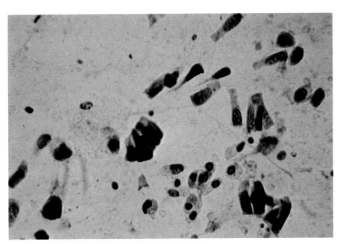

14.105

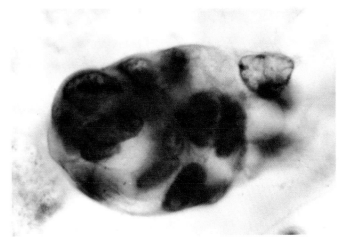

14.107

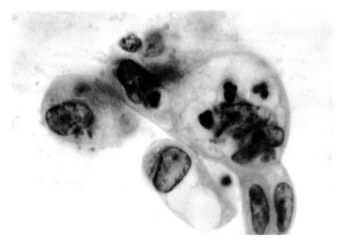

14.104

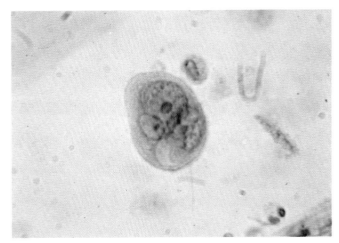

14.106

14.108

Figs. 14.109 and 14.110. Adenocarcinoma of the pancreas; small groups of malignant cells (Pap stain). × 1,000.

Fig. 14.111. Adenocarcinoma of the gallbladder; hyperchromatic isolated malignant cells (Pap stain). × 1,000.

Figs. 14.112 to 14.114. Microscopy of bile; typical cholesterol crystals and calcium bilirubinate granules.

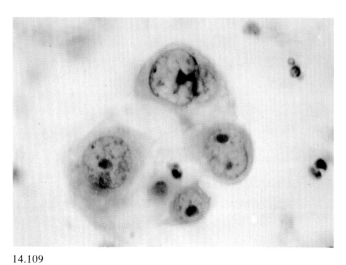

14.109

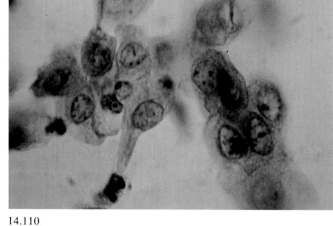

14.110

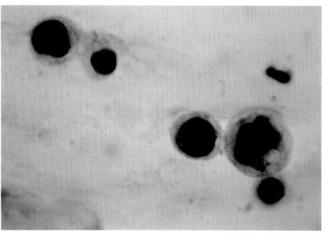

14.111

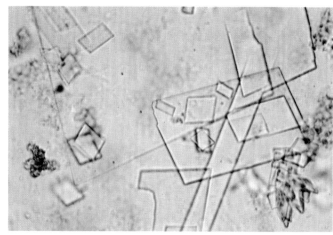

14.112

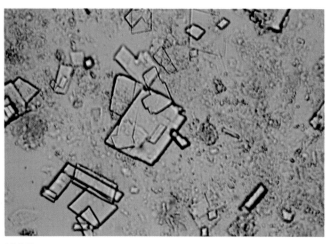

14.113

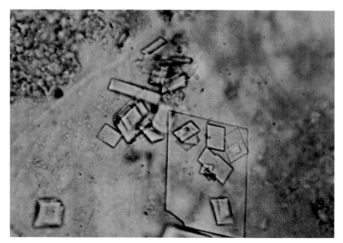

14.114

101

Figs. 14.115 to 14.118. Microscopy of bile; *Giardia lamblia* (Pap stain). × 1,000.

Fig. 14.119. Normal colon histology; superficial epithelium (hematoxylin and eosin stain). × 100.

Fig. 14.120. Normal colon; superficial epithelial cells (Pap stain). × 1,000.

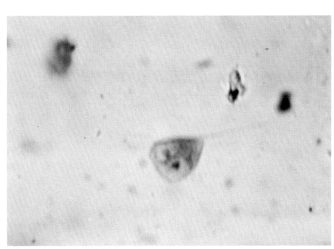

14.115

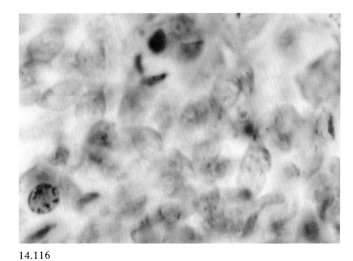

14.116

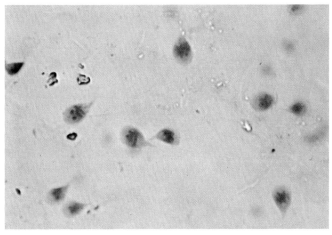

14.117

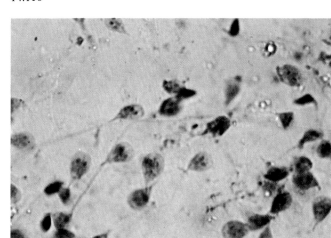

14.118

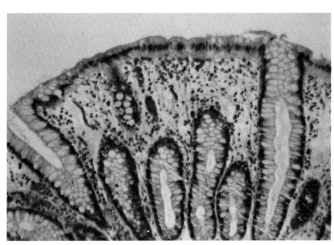

14.119

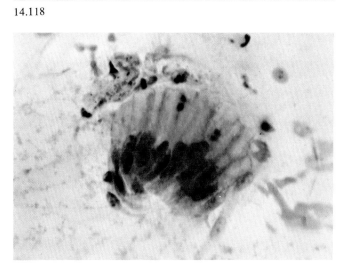

14.120

Fig. 14.121. Chronic ulcerative colitis histology; atypical epithelial changes and carcinoma in situ (hematoxylin and eosin stain). × 100. This figure should be viewed with the right edge at the top.

Fig. 14.122. Chronic ulcerative colitis histology; cytological changes in atypical glands (hematoxylin and eosin stain). × 400.

Fig. 14.123. Chronic ulcerative colitis histology; area of carcinoma in situ (hematoxylin and eosin stain). × 100.

Figs. 14.124 and 14.125. Chronic ulcerative colitis; examples of "bland" cells (Pap stain). × 1,000.

Fig. 14.126. Chronic ulcerative colitis; examples of "active" cells (Pap stain). × 1,000.

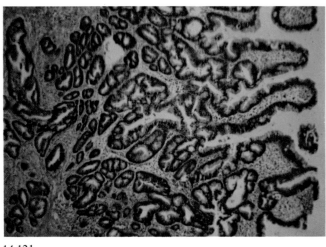

14.121

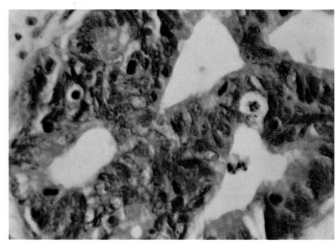

14.122

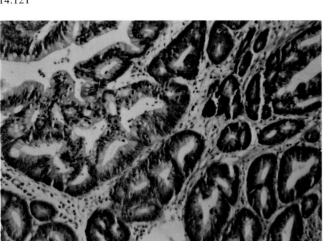

14.123

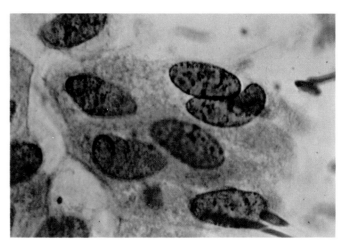

14.124

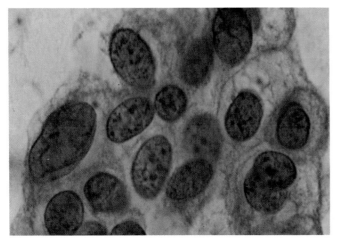

14.125

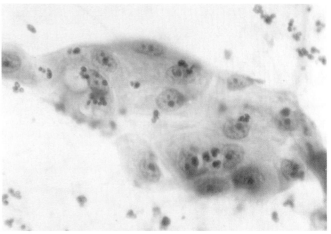

14.126

Figs. 14.127 and 14.128.
Chronic ulcerative colitis;
examples of "active" cells
(Pap stain). × 1,000.

Figs. 14.129 to 14.132.
Chronic ulcerative colitis;
advanced degree of cellular
atypia (Pap stain). × 1,000.

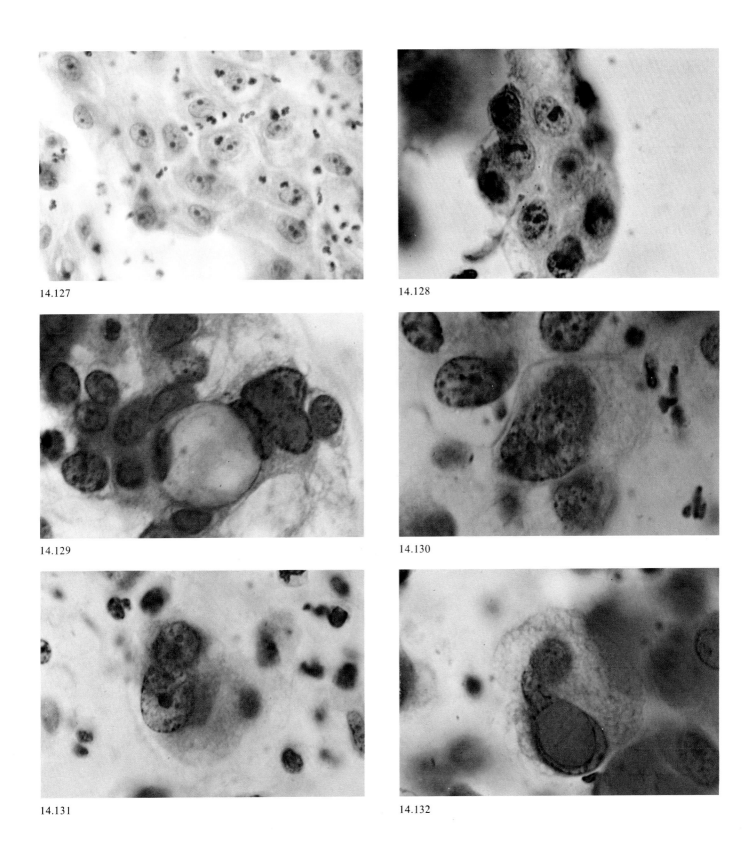

14.127

14.128

14.129

14.130

14.131

14.132

104

Figs. 14.133 to 14.136. Chronic ulcerative colitis; nonepithelial atypical cells (Pap stain). × 1,000.

Fig. 14.137. Irradiation proctitis; group of atypical epithelial cells (Pap stain). × 400.

Fig. 14.138. Adenocarcinoma of the colon; isolated cells and groups of malignant cells with prominent red nucleoli (Pap stain). × 1,000.

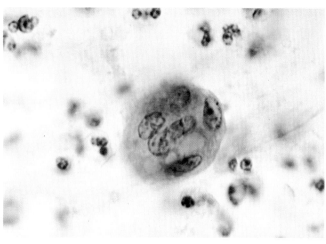

14.133

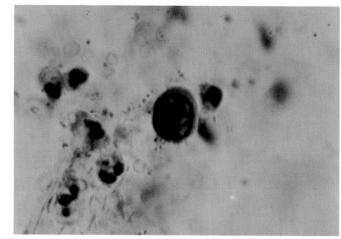

14.134

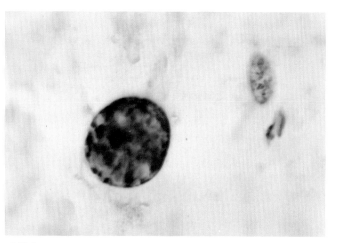

14.135

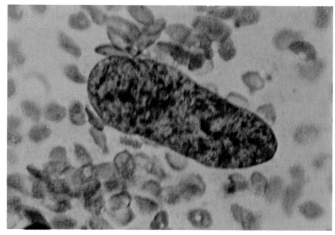

14.136

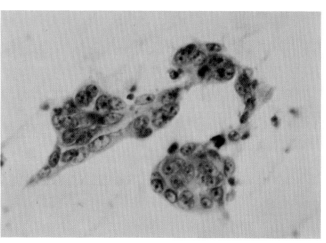

14.137

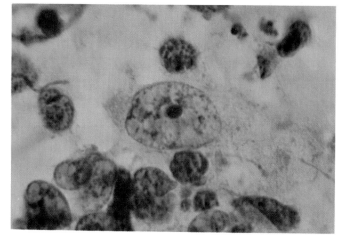

14.138

Figs. 14.139 to 14.144. Adenocarcinoma of the colon; isolated cells and groups of malignant cells with prominent red nucleoli (Pap stain). × 1,000.

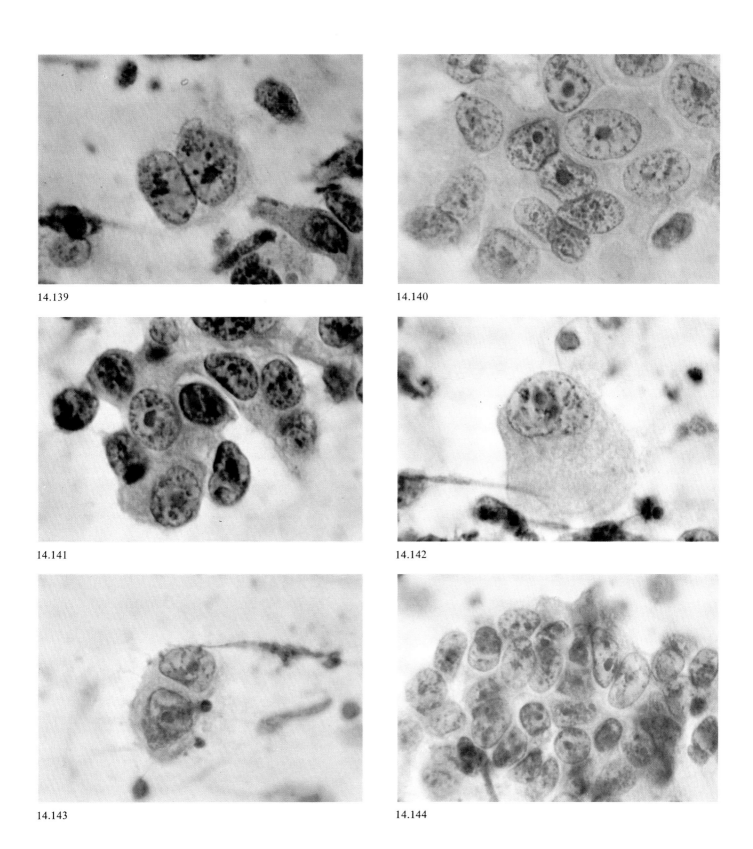

14.139

14.140

14.141

14.142

14.143

14.144

Fig. 14.145. Adenocarcinoma of the colon; isolated cells and groups of malignant cells with prominent red nucleoli (Pap stain). × 1,000.

Figs. 14.146 and 14.147. Adenocarcinoma of the colon; anaplastic cells with irregularly shaped nuclei (Pap stain). × 1,000.

Figs. 14.148 to 14.150. Adenocarcinoma of the colon; large anaplastic cells (Pap stain). × 1,000.

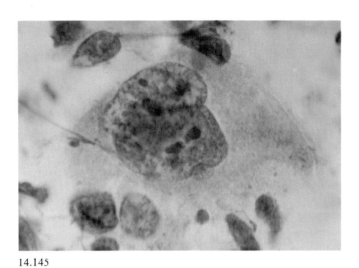

14.145

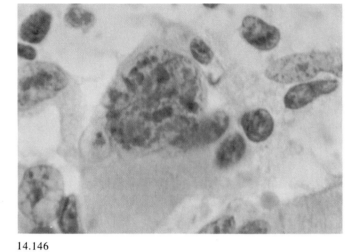

14.146

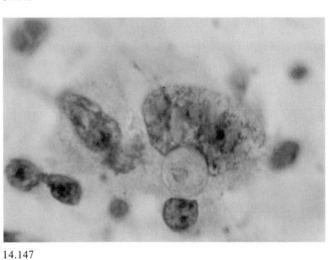

14.147

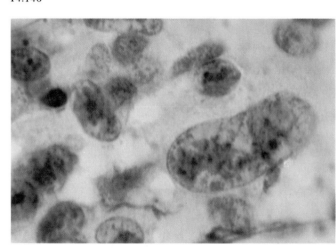

14.148

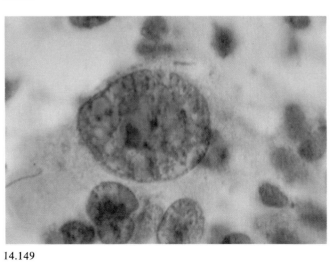

14.149

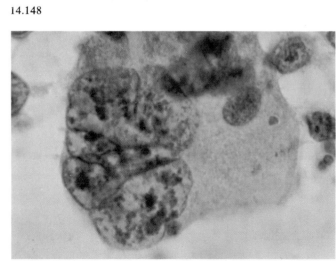

14.150

107

Figs. 14.151 and 14.152. Adenocarcinoma of the colon; large anaplastic cells (Pap stain). × 1,000.

Figs. 14.153 to 14.155. Adenocarcinoma of the colon; groups of malignant cells, some of which are signet-ring cells (Pap stain). × 1,000.

Fig. 14.156. Acridine-Orange technique; normal gastric epithelial cells. × 400.

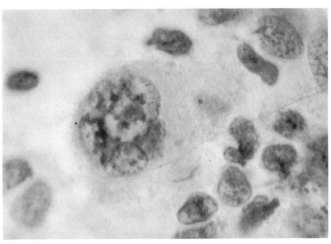

14.151

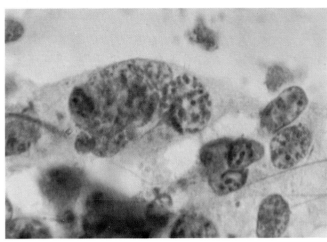

14.152

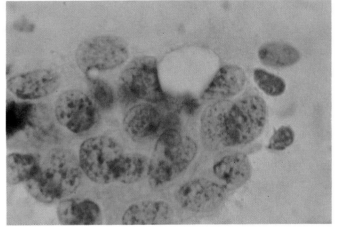

14.153

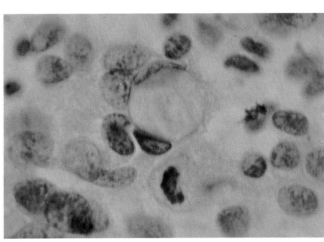

14.154

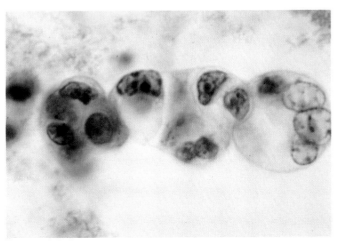

14.155

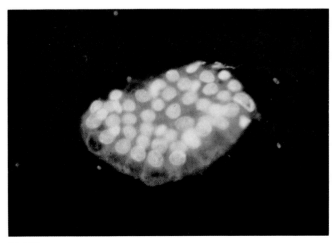

14.156

108

Figs. 14.157 and 14.158. Acridine-Orange technique; normal gastric epithelial cells. × 400.

Figs. 14.159 to 14.161. Acridine-Orange technique; slightly atypical cells from cases of benign gastric ulcer. × 400.

Fig. 14.162. Acridine-Orange technique; squamous cell carcinoma of the esophagus. × 400.

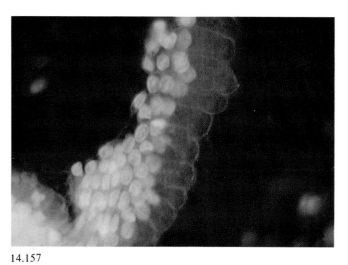

14.157

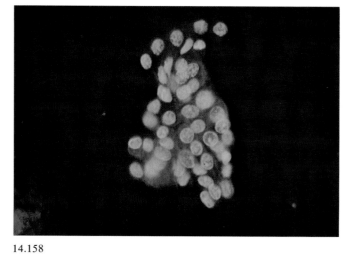

14.158

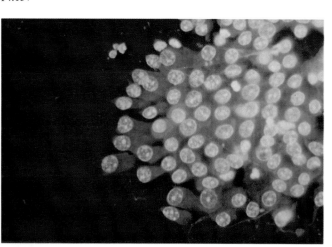

14.159

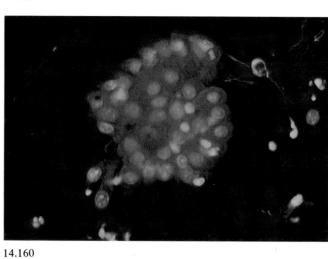

14.160

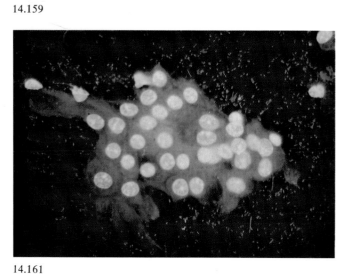

14.161

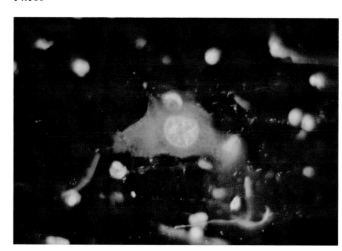

14.162

109

Fig. 14.163. Acridine-Orange technique; squamous cell carcinoma of the esophagus. × 400.

Figs. 14.164 to 14.167. Acridine-Orange technique; adenocarcinoma of the stomach; large groups of malignant cells. × 400.

Fig. 14.168. Acridine-Orange technique; high-power view of malignant cells in adenocarcinoma of the stomach, showing excellent morphological detail. × 1,000.

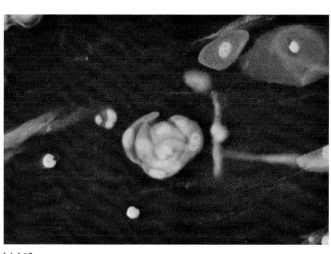

14.163

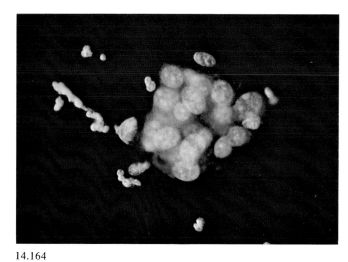

14.164

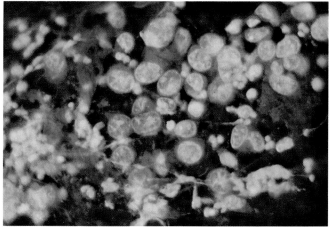

14.165

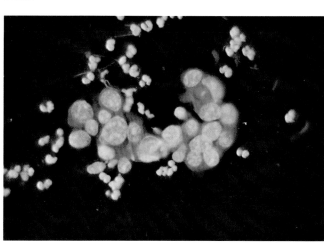

14.166

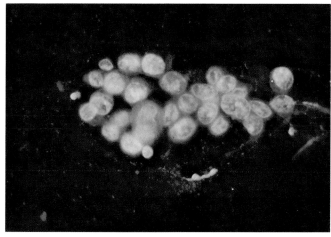

14.167

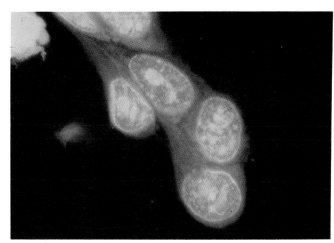

14.168

Figs. 14.169 to 14.172. Acridine-Orange technique; high-power view of malignant cells in adenocarcinoma of the stomach, showing excellent morphological detail. × 1,000.

Fig. 14.173. Shorr's technique; cytology from a case of gastric ulcer. × 500.

Fig. 14.174. Shorr's technique; cytology from a case of adenocarcinoma of the stomach.

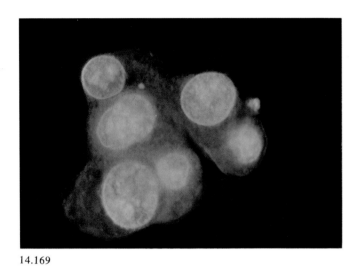

14.169

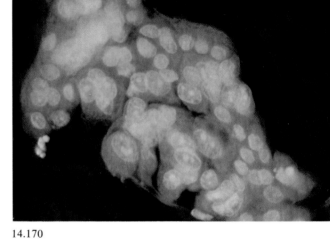

14.170

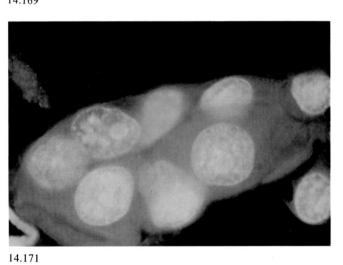

14.171

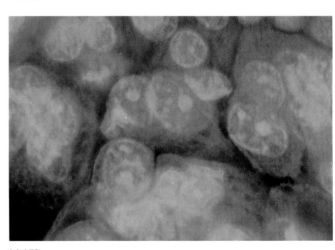

14.172

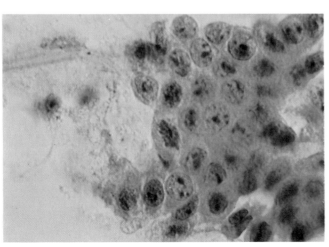

14.173

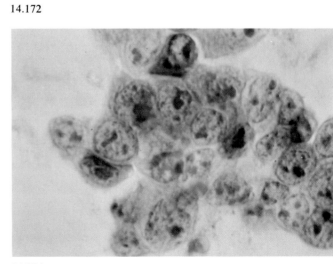

14.174

Fig. 14.175. Shorr's technique; cytology from a case of adenocarcinoma of the stomach.

Figs. 14.176 to 14.180. May-Grunwald-Giemsa technique; cytology from several cases of adenocarcinoma of the stomach. (These pictures were provided by Dr. T. Kasugai and Dr. S. Kobayashi, from Nagoya, Japan.)

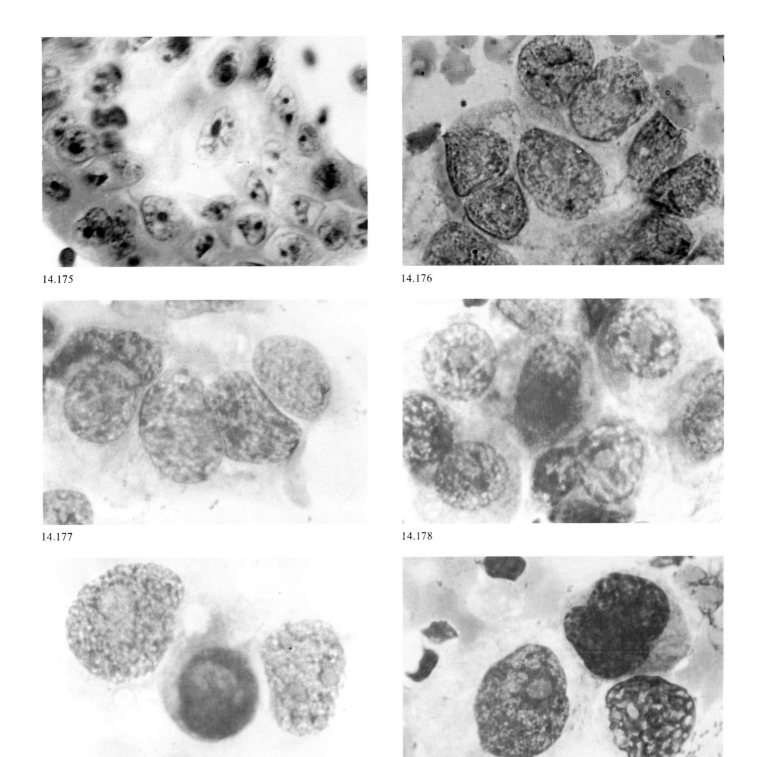

14.175

14.176

14.177

14.178

14.179

14.180

112

Figs. 14.181 and 14.182. May-Grunwald-Giemsa technique; cytology of another case of adenocarcinoma of the stomach.

Fig. 15.1. Group of lymphocytes, in a case of gastric lymphoma (Pap stain). × 1,000.

Figs. 15.2 and 15.3. Isolated large immature lymphocytes, in a case of gastric lymphoma (Pap stain). × 1,000.

Fig. 15.4. Large immature lymphoid cells, from a case of gastric lymphoma (May-Grunwald-Giemsa technique). × 1,250. (This picture was provided by Drs. T. Kasugai and S. Kobayashi, from Nagoya, Japan.)

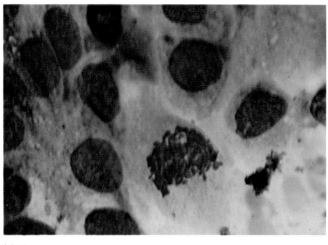

14.181

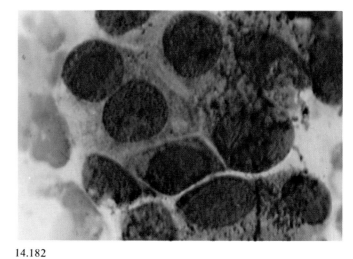

14.182

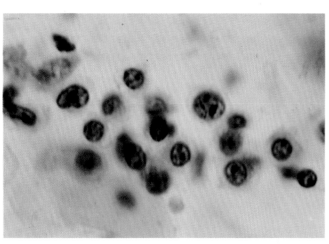

15.1

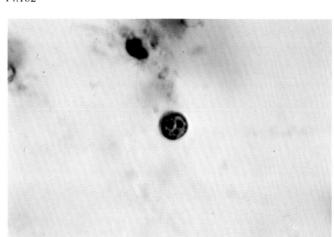

15.2

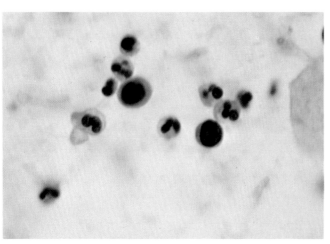

15.3

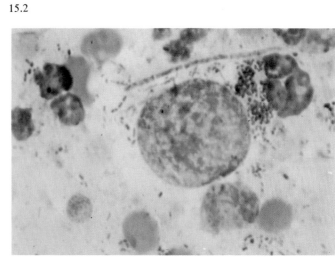

15.4

113

Fig. 15.5. Large immature lymphoid cells, from a case of gastric lymphoma (May-Grunwald-Giemsa technique). × 1,250. (This picture was provided by Drs. T. Kasugai and S. Kobayashi, from Nagoya, Japan.)

Figs. 15.6 and 15.7. Reticulum type cells, from a case of gastric lymphoma (Pap stain). × 1,000.

Figs. 15.8 and 15.9. Groups of isolated reticulum type cells, from a case of gastric lymphoma (May-Grunwald-Giemsa technique). × 1,000. (This case was studied by us courtesy of Drs. Kasugai and Kobayashi, from Nagoya, Japan.)

Fig. 15.10. Reticulum type of cells, from a case of gastric lymphoma (Pap stain). × 1,000.

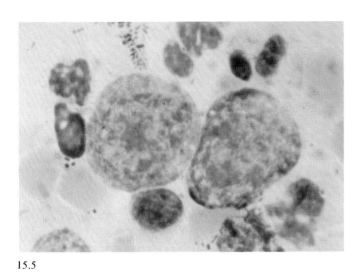

15.5

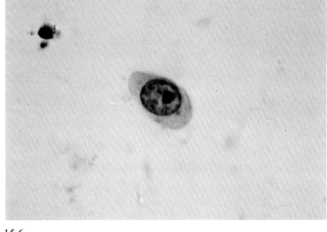

15.6

15.7

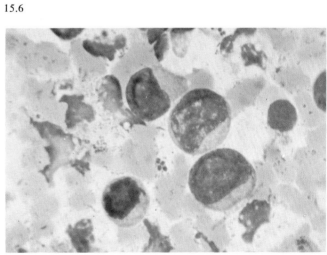

15.8

15.9

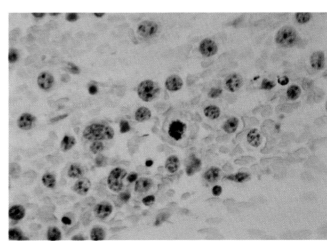

15.10

114

Figs. 15.11 to 15.13. Reticulum type of cells, from a case of gastric lymphoma (Pap stain). × 1,000.

Fig. 15.14. Large reticulum cell from a case of gastric lymphoma (Pap stain). × 1,000.

Figs. 15.15 and 15.16. Reed-Sternberg cells from two cases of Hodgkin's disease involving the stomach (Pap stain). × 1,000.

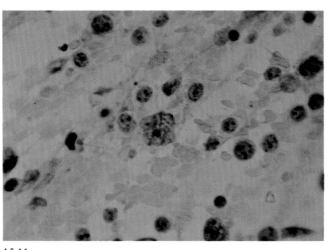

15.11

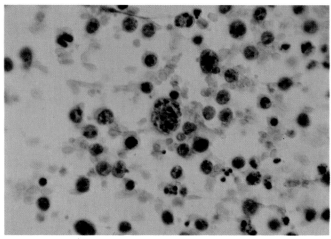

15.12

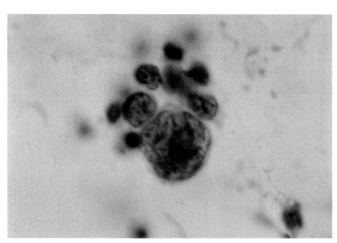

15.13

15.14

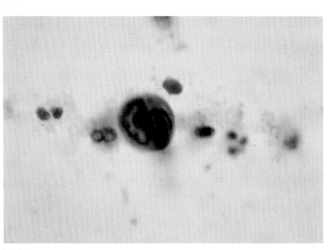

15.15

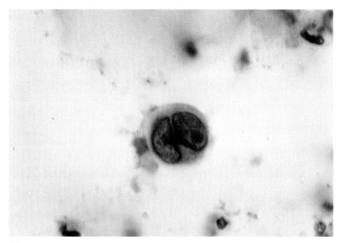

15.16

115

Figs. 15.17 and 15.18. Loosely arranged clusters of malignant cells, in a case of gastric lymphoma (Pap stain). × 1,000.

Figs. 15.19 to 15.21. May-Grunwald-Giemsa staining of material from same case shown in figs. 15.17 and 15.18. Isolated reticulum type of malignant cells, some in mitosis. × 1,000.

Fig. 15.22. Gastric reactive lymphoreticular hyperplasia ("pseudolymphoma"). Pools of lymphocytes, with some plasma cells. × 1,000.

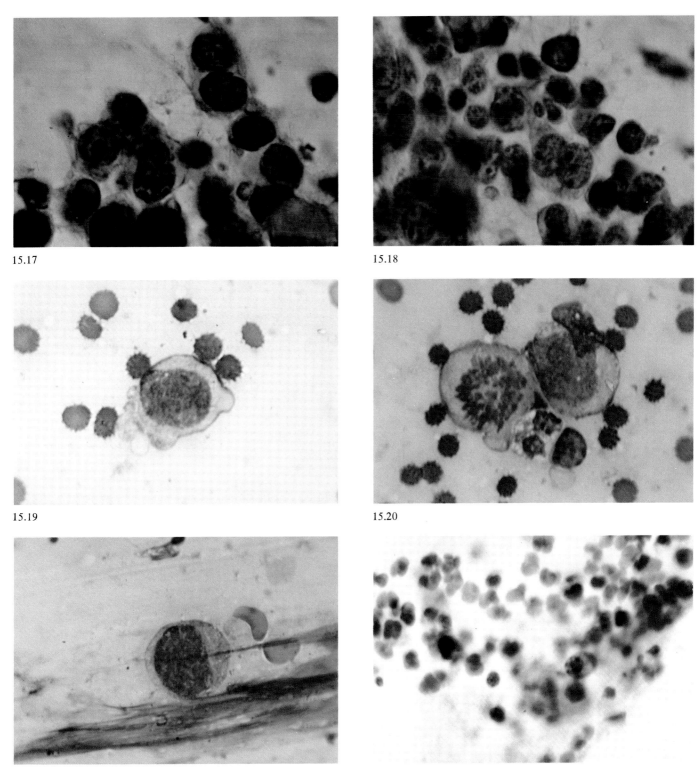

15.17

15.18

15.19

15.20

15.21

15.22

Fig. 15.23. Gastric reactive lymphoreticular hyperplasia ("pseudolymphoma"). Pools of lymphocytes, with some plasma cells. × 1,000.

Figs. 15.24 to 15.26. Plasma cells in a case of histiocytic lymphoma of the stomach (May-Grunwald-Giemsa stain). × 1,000.

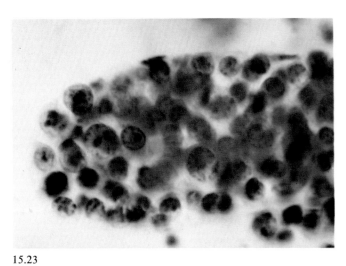

15.23

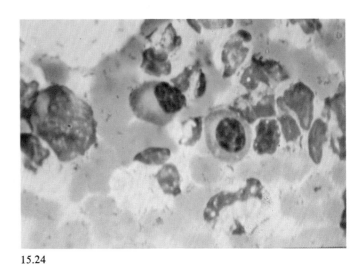

15.24

15.25

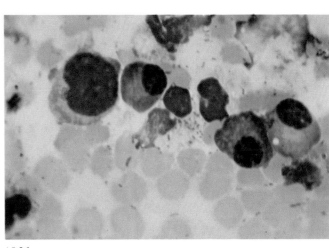

15.26

References

1. Ackerman, N. B. 1967. An evaluation of gastric cytology: Results of a nationwide survey. *J. Chron. Dis.* 20:621–26.

2. Allen, A. R., and Fullmer, C. D. 1969. Hypochromic carcinomas and criteria of hypochromic neoplastic cells: Presentation of a case. *Acta Cytol.* 13:485–87.

3. Andersen, H. A.; McDonald, J. R.; and Olsen, A. M. 1949. Cytological diagnosis of malignant lesions of the esophagus and cardia of stomach. *Proc. Mayo Clin.* 24:245–53; *Minnesota Med.* 32:1181–85.

4. Andrew, W., and Collings, C. K. 1946. Lymphocytes within the cells of intestinal epithelium in man. *Anat. Rec.* 96:445–57.

5. Anthonisen, P., and Riis, P. 1962. Cytology of colonic secretion in proctosigmoidal disease. *Acta Med. Scand.* 172:375–81.

6. Ariga, K. 1967. Statistics of mass survey of the stomach in 1966. *Gastric Cancer and Mass Survey* 14:103–6 (in Japanese).

7. Aronson, A. R., and Darling, D. R. 1959. Carcinoma at the margin of the gastrojejunostomy stoma: Review of the literature and report of a case. *Gastroenterology* 36:686–90.

8. Atkin, N. B. 1964. Nuclear size in carcinoma of the cervix: Its relation to DNA content and prognosis. *Cancer* 17:1391–99.

9. ———. 1969. Variant nuclear types in gynecologic tumors: Observations on squashes and smears. *Acta Cytol,* 13:569–75.

10. Ayre, J. E., and Oren, B. G. 1953. A new rapid method for stomach cancer diagnosis: The gastric brush. *Cancer* 6:1177–81.

11. ———. 1957. Colon brush: A new diagnostic procedure for cancer of the lower bowel. *Amer. J. Dig. Dis.* 2:74–80.

12. Bader, G. M., and Papanicolaou, G. N. 1952. Application of cytology in diagnosis of cancer of rectum, sigmoid and descending colon. *Cancer* 5:307–14.

13. Barton, K. B.; Prolla, J. C.; and Kirsner, J. B. 1965. Preliminary cytochemical studies of mucosal surface cells in ulcerative colitis. *Acta Cytol.* 9:239–43.

14. Beale, L. S. 1858. *The microscope in medicine.* 2d ed. London: J. and A. Churchill.

15. Bennington, J. L.; Porus, R.; Ferguson, B.; and Hannon, G. 1968. Cytology of gastric sarcoid: Report of a case. *Acta Cytol.* 12:30–36.

16. Bercovitz, Z. 1941. Studies in cellular exudates of bowel discharges. III. The diagnostic significance of cellular exudate studies in chronic bowel disorders. *Ann. Intern Med.* 14:1323–40.

17. Berkowitz, D.; Cooney, P.; and Bralow, S. P. 1959. Carcinoma of the stomach appearing after previous gastric surgery for benign ulcer disease. *Gastroenterology* 36:691–97.

18. Berry, A. V.; Livni, N. M.; and Epstein, N. 1969. Some observations on cell morphology in the cytodiagnosis of endometrial carcinoma. *Acta Cytol.* 13:530–33.

19. Berry, T. J.; Lee, T. C.; and Coffey, R. J. 1959. Carcinoma arising in the gastric stump following gastric resection for benign ulceration. *Amer. Surg.* 25:353.

20. Bertalanffy, F. D. 1961. Diagnostic reliability of the Acridine-Orange fluorescence microscope method for cytodiagnosis of cancer. *Cancer Res.* 21:422–26.

21. ———. 1962. Evaluation of the Acridine-Orange fluorescence microscope method for cytodiagnosis of cancer. *Ann. N.Y. Acad. Sci.* 93:715–50.

22. Bessis, M. 1956. *Cytology of the blood and blood-forming organs.* New York: Grune and Stratton.

23. Blank, W. A., and Steinberg, A. H. 1951. Cytologic diagnosis of malignancies of the lower bowel and rectum. *Amer. J. Surg.* 81:127–31.

24. Block, D. E., and Lancaster, G. R. 1964. Adenocarcinoma of the cardioesophageal junction. *Arch. Surg.* 88:852–59.

25. Boas, I. 1897. Diagnostik und Therapie der Magenkrankheiten. Vol. I, part 4. Leipzig; Georg Thieme.

26. Bockus, H. L. 1965. Diagnostic studies in affections of gall bladder and bile ducts. II. Biliary drainage procedures and other laboratory aids. In *Gastroenterology,* 2d ed., ed. H. L. Bockus, vol. 3, chap. 109, Philadelphia: W. B. Saunders.

27. Bockus, H. L.; Lopusniak, M. S.; and Tachdjian, V. 1965. Diagnostic procedures in the study of pancreatic disorders. I. Laboratory procedures. *Gastroenterology,* 2d ed., ed. H. L. Bockus, vol. 3, chap. 123. Philadelphia: W. B. Saunders.

28. Bockus, H. L.; Shay, H.; Willard, J. H.; and Pessel, J. F. 1931. Comparison of biliary drainage and cholecystography in gallstone diagnosis, with special

reference to bile microscopy. *J.A.M.A.* 96:311.

29. Boddington, M. M., and Truelove, S. C. 1956. Abnormal epithelial cells in ulcerative colitis. *Brit. Med. J.* 1:1318–21.

30. Boen, S. T. 1957. Changes in nuclei of squamous epithelial cells in pernicious anemia. *Acta Med. Scand.* 159:425–31.

31. Boon, T. H.; Schade, R. O. K.; Middleton, G. D.; and Reece, M. F. 1964. An attempt at presymptomatic diagnosis of gastric carcinoma in pernicious anemia. *Gut* 5:269–70.

32. Bowden, L., and Papanicolaou, G. N. 1959. Exfoliated pancreatic cancer cells in the duct of Wirsung. *Ann. Surg.* 150:296–98.

33. ———. 1960. The diagnosis of pancreatic cancer by cytologic study of duodenal secretions. *Acta Un. Int. Cancr.* 16:398–404.

34. Brandborg, L. L.; Taniguchi, L.; and Rubin, C. E. 1961. Is exfoliative cytology practical for more general use in the diagnosis of gastric cancer? *Cancer* 14:1074–80.

35. Brandborg, L. L.; Tankersley, C. B.; and Uyeda, F. 1969. "Low" versus "high" concentration chymotrypsin in gastric exfoliative cytology. *Gastroenterology* 57:500–505.

36. Brandborg, L. L., and Wenger, J. 1968. Cytological examination in gastrointestinal tract disease. *Med. Clin. N. Amer.* 52:1315–28.

37. Bruinsma, A. H. 1957. The value of cytology in the early diagnosis of carcinoma of the esophagus and stomach (making use of the Papanicolaou gastric balloon and its modifications). Thesis, Utrecht.

38. Burdman, D.; Garret, M.; and Benninghoff, D. L. 1969. Comparative cytomorphology of irradiation atypia and chemically induced carcinoma in the mouse cervix. *Acta Cytol.* 13:620–33.

39. Burkalow, P.; Medak, H.; McGrew, E. A.; and Tiecke, R. 1969. The cytology of vesicular conditions affecting the oral mucosa. 2. Keratosis follicularis. *Acta Cytol.* 13:407–15.

40. Burnett, W.; MacFarlane, P. S.; Scott, S. D.; and Kay, A. W. 1960. Carcinoma of the stomach: An evaluation of diagnostic methods including exfoliative cytology. *Brit. Med. J.* 1:753–55.

41. Byrnes, W. W., and Lemon, H. M. 1954. The cytologic diagnosis of cancer of the pancreas and biliary tract. In *Transactions, Second Annual Meeting, Inter-Society Cytology Council,* Boston, 12–13 November, 1954.

42. Cabre-Fiol, V. 1953. Procedimiento de obtención de muestras para citologia endogástrica. *Rev. Esp. Enferm. Apar. Dig.* 12:186.

43. Cabre-Fiol, V., and Olo-Garcia, R. 1962. Citodiagnóstico de las neoplasias gástricas malignas por biopsia exfoliativa. *Rev. Esp. Enferm. Apar. Dig.* 21:571.

44. Cabre-Fiol, V.; Olo-Garcia, R.; and Vilardell, F. 1958. Five years of cytologic diagnosis of gastric cancer by "exfoliative biopsy" (abstr). In *Proceedings of the World Congress on Gastroenterology,* 2:1006. Baltimore: Williams and Wilkins.

45. Cameron, A. B. 1960. A cytologic method of diagnosis of carcinoma of the colon. *Dis. Colon Rectum* 3:230–36.

46. Cameron, A. B., and Thabet, R. J. 1959. Recovery of malignant cells from enema returns in carcinoma of colon. *Surg. Forum* 10:30–33.

47. Cantor, M. O. 1949. *Intestinal intubation.* Springfield, Ill.: Charles C. Thomas.

48. Cantrell, E. G. 1968. An evaluation of cytology in the diagnosis of carcinoma of the stomach. M.D. diss., Cambridge.

49. ———. 1969. Why use gastric cytology? *Gut* 10: 763–66.

50. Capos, N. J., and Hyman, S. 1961. Cancer in the residual stomach after gastric resection for duodenal ulcer. *J.A.M.A.* 177:448.

51. Caspersson, T., and Santesson, L. 1942. Studies on protein metabolism in the cells of epithelial tumors. *Acta Radiol.,* suppl. 46.

52. Chiampo, L., and Rigamonti, P. P. 1962. Possibilita diagnostiche della micròscopia a' fluorescenza con colorazione all'arancio di acridina nella citologia esfoliativa gastrica. *Arch. Ital. Mal. Appar. Dig.* 29: 288–300.

53. Coffey, R. J., and Cardenas, F. 1964. Clinical features of carcinoma of the gastric stump following gastric resection for benign peptic ulcer. *Amer. J. Gastroent.* 42:77–84.

54. Coleman, D. V. 1969. A case of tuberculosis of the cervix. *Acta Cytol.* 14:104–7.

55. Collins, E. N. 1939. The indications for duodenal drainage: Its relation to cholecystography. *Cleveland Clin. Quart.* 6:185.

56. Coman, D. R. 1944. Decreased mutual adhesiveness, property of cells from squamous cell carcinoma. *Cancer Res.* 4:625–29.

57. Cone, C. D., Jr. 1969. Autosynchrony and self-induced mitosis in sarcoma cell networks. *Acta Cytol.* 13:576–82.

58. Cooper, W. A., and Papanicolaou, G. N. 1953. Balloon technique in the cytological diagnosis of gastric cancer. *J.A.M.A.* 151:10–14.

59. Dawson, I. M. P., and Pryse-Davies, J. 1959. The development of carcinoma of the large intestine in ulcerative colitis. *Brit. J. Surg.* 47:113–28.

60. Debray, C.; Housset, P.; Martin, E.; Bourdais, J. P.; and Nicolaidis, C. L. 1962. A new direct-vision biopsy gastroscope. *Gut* 3:273–76.

61. Diamond, J. S., and Siegel, S. A. 1940. The secretin test in the diagnosis of pancreatic disease, with a report of 130 tests. *Amer. J. Dig. Dis.* 7:435–45.

62. Dornberger, G. R.; Comfort, M. W.; Wollaeger, E. E.; and Power, M. H. 1948. Pancreatic function as measured by analysis of duodenal contents before and after stimulation with secretin. *Gastroenterology* 11:701.

63. Dreiling, D. A. 1957. The pancreatic secretion in the malabsorption syndrome and related malnutrition states. *J. Mount Sinai Hosp. N.Y.* 24:243.

64. ———. 1951. Studies in pancreatic function. IV. The use of the secretin test in the diagnosis of tumors in and about the pancreas. *Gastroenterology* 18:185–96.

65. Dreiling, D. A., and Hollander, F. 1950. Studies in pancreatic function. II. Statistical study of pancreatic secretion following secretin in patients without pancreatic disease. *Gastroenterology* 15:620.

66. Dreiling, D. A.; Janowitz, H. D.; and Perrier, C. V. 1964. *Pancreatic inflammatory disease: A physiologic approach.* New York: Hoeber Medical Div. of Harper and Row.

67. Dreiling, D. A.; Nieburgs, H. E.; and Janowitz, H. D. 1960. The combined secretin and cytology test in the diagnosis of pancreatic and biliary tract cancer. *Med. Clin. N. Amer.* 44:801–15.

68. Einhorn, M. 1921. Cases of gallbladder lesions simulating other affections of the digestive tract. *Med. Rec.* 100:1015.

69. Fawcett, D. W. 1966. *An atlas of fine structure: The cell; its organelles and inclusions.* Philadelphia: W. B. Saunders.

70. Fennessy, J. J.; Sparberg, M. B.; and Kirsner, J. B. 1968. Radiological findings in carcinoma of the colon complicating chronic ulcerative colitis. *Gut* 9:388–97.

71. Fischman, M., and Terzano, G. 1955. Gastric cytology by the abrasive balloon method. *Gastroenterology* 29:1046–54.

72. ———. 1958. Citologia gástrica: Método del balón abrasivo de Panico, Papanicolaou y Cooper. *Acta Un. Int. Cancr.* 14:923–32.

73. Forni, A. M.; Koss, L. G.; and Geller, W. 1964. Cytological study of the effect of cyclophosphamide on the epithelium of the urinary bladder in man. *Cancer* 17:1348–55.

74. Foushee, J. H. S.; Kalnins, Z. A.; Dixon, F. R.; Girsh, S.; Morehead, R. P.; O'Brien, T. F.; Pribor, H.; and Tattory, C. 1969. Gastric cytology: Evaluation of methods and results in 1,670 cases. *Acta Cytol.* 13:399–406.

75. Fridman, E. G. 1963. Cancer of resected stomach: Analysis of 194 cases. *Acta Un. Int. Cancr.* 19:1257–60.

76. Fuchs, B. J.; Duke, P. S.; Schwinn, C. P.; and Demopoulos, H. B. 1968. Cytologic study of the effects of L-cysteine on pigmented mouse melanoma cells and heart cells in tissue culture, with special reference to nuclear lobulation. *Acta Cytol.* 12:325–31.

77. Fukuda, T.; Shida, S.; Takita, T.; and Sawada, Y. 1967. Cytologic diagnosis of early gastric cancer by the endoscope method with gastrofiberscope. *Acta Cytol.* 11:456–59.

78. Fullmer, C. D.; Short, J. G.; Allen, A.; and Walker, K. 1969. Proposed classification for bronchial epithelial cell abnormalities in the category of dyskaryosis. *Acta Cytol.* 13:459–71.

79. Galambos, J. T. 1962. Cytologic examination of benign colonic lesions. *Acta Cytol.* 6:148–54.

80. Galambos, J. T., and Klayman, M. I. 1955. The clinical value of colonic exfoliative cytology in the diagnosis of cancer beyond the reach of the proctoscope. *Surg. Gynec. Obstet.* 101:673–79.

81. Galambos, J. T.; Massey, B. W.; Klayman, M. I.; and Kirsner, J. B. 1956. Exfoliative cytology in chronic ulcerative colitis. *Cancer* 9:152–59.

82. Gardner, F. N. 1956. Observations on the cytology of gastric epithelium in tropical sprue. *J. Lab. Clin. Med.* 47:529–39.

References

83. Gatch, W. D. 1957. Degree of adhesiveness of cancer cells and its relation to cancer spread. *Arch. Surg.* 74:753–57.

84. Gephart, T., and Graham, R. M. 1959. The cellular detection of carcinoma of the esophagus. *Surg. Gynec. Obstet.* 108:75–82.

85. Gerstenberg, E.; Albrecht, A.; Krentz, K.; and Voth, H. 1965. Das Magenstumpfkarzinom eine Spätkomplikation des operierten Magens? *Deutsch. Med. Wschr.* 90:2185.

86. Gibbs, G. E. 1950. Secretin test with bilumen gastroduodenal drainage in infants and children. *Pediatrics* 5:941–46.

87. Gibbs, D. D. 1962. Carcinoma in the gastric remnant after partial gastrectomy for benign ulceration. *Gut* 3:322–26.

88. ———. 1968. *Exfoliative cytology of the stomach.* New York: Appleton-Century-Crofts; London; Butterworth.

89. Go, V. L. W.; Hofmann, A. F.; and Summerskill, W. H. J. 1970. Simultaneous measurements of total pancreatic, biliary, and gastric outputs in man using a perfusion technique. *Gastroenterology* 58:321–28.

90. Gold, P. 1967. Circulating antibodies against carcinoembyronic antigens of the human digestive system. *Cancer* 20:1663–67.

91. Goldb, M. 1947. An appraisal of the value of diagnostic biliary drainage. *Amer. J. Dig. Dis.* 14:263.

92. Goldgraber, M. B. 1956. The response of esophageal cancer to irradiation: A serial study of two cases. *Gastroenterology* 30:618–24.

93. Goldgraber, M. B., and Kirsner, J. B. 1964. Carcinoma of the colon in ulcerative colitis. *Cancer* 17:657–65.

94. Goldgraber, M. B.; Rubin, C. E.; and Owens, F. J. 1953. The cytological diagnosis of duodenal sarcoma (polymorphic reticulosarcoma). *Ann. Intern. Med.* 39:1316–22.

95. Goldstein, H., and Ventzke, L. E. 1968. Value of exfoliative cytology in pancreatic carcinoma. *Gut* 9:316–18.

96. Grable, E.; Zamcheck, N.; Jankelson, O.; and Shipp, F. 1957. Nuclear size of cells in normal stomachs, in gastric atrophy and in gastric cancer. *Gastroenterology* 32:1104–12.

97. Graham, R. M. 1963. *The cytologic diagnosis of cancer.* 2d ed. Philadelphia: W. B. Saunders.

98. Graham, R. M., and Rheault, M. H. 1954. Characteristic cellular changes in epithelial cells in pernicious anemia. *J. Lab. Clin. Med.* 43:235–45.

99. Graham, R. M.; Ulfelder, H.; and Green, T. H. 1948. The cytologic method as an aid in the diagnosis of gastric carcinoma. *Surg. Gynec. Obstet.* 86:257–59.

100. Gross, J. B.; Comfort, M. W.; Wollaeger, E. E.; and Power, M. H. 1950. External pancreatic function in primary parenchymatous hepatic disease as measured by analysis of duodenal contents, before and after stimulation with secretin. *Gastroenterology* 16:151–61.

101. Grubb, C., and Crabbé, J. G. S. 1961. Fluorescence microscopy in exfoliative cytology. *Brit. J. Cancer* 15:483–88.

102. Gutmann, R. A.; Bertrand, I.; and Peristiany, T. J. 1939. *Le cancer de l'estomac au début.* Paris: G. Doin et Cie.

103. Hampton, J. M.; Bacon, H. E.; and Myers, J. 1962. A simplified method for the diagnosis of cancer of the colon by exfoliative cytology. *Dis. Colon Rectum* 5:145–47.

104. Hayashi, K., and Sugiura, Y. 1966. Direct-vision biopsy and cytology. *Gastroent. Endosc.* (*Tokyo*) 8:37–39 (in Japanese).

105. Hayashida, T., amd Kidokoro, T. 1969. End results of early gastric cancer collected from twenty-two institutions. *Stomach Intest.* (*Tokyo*) 4:1077–85.

106. Heindenreich, A. 1961. Rectocolic exfoliative cytology. *Prensa Med. Argent.* 47:2009–19.

107. Hemmeter, J. 1889. The early diagnosis of cancer of the stomach. *Med. Rec.* (*N.Y.*) 46:577.

108. Henning, N., and Witte, S. 1951. Untersuchungen zur Cytologie des Duodenalinhalts. *Deutsch. Arch. Klin. Med.* 198:91.

109. ———. 1952. Über eine neue Methode zur Zytodiagnostik der Magenkrankheiten. *Deutsch. Med. Wschr.* 77:1–4.

110. ———. 1970. *Atlas of gastrointestinal cytodiagnosis.* 2d ed. Stuttgart: Georg Thieme.

111. Henning, N.; Witte, S.; and Bressel, D. 1960. Über den Befund von Leberzellen in Duodenalinhalt und seinen Diagnostischen. *Wert. Med. Klin.* 55:962.

112. Henning, N.; Witte, S.; and Bressel, D. 1964. The cytologic diagnosis of tumors of the upper gastro-

intestinal tract (esophagus, stomach, duodenum). *Acta Cytol.* 8:121–30.

113. Hershenson, L. M.; Lerch, V.; and Hershenson, M. A. 1958. Esophageal cytology by a gauge-sponge smear technique. *J.A.M.A.* 168:1871–75.

114. Hinton, J. M. 1966. Risk of malignant change in ulcerative colitis. *Gut* 7:427–32.

115. Hirschowitz, B. I.; Curtiss, L. E.; Peters, C. W.; and Pollard, H. M. 1958. Demonstration of a new gastroscope. *Gastroenterology* 35:50–53.

116. Hoffmann, R. G. 1963. Statistics in the practice of medicine. *J.A.M.A.* 185:864–73.

117. Humphreys, E. A.; Wolff, R. A.; and Mlecko, L. M. 1968. "Scrape" cytology of the esophagus and stomach. *Gastroint. Endosc.* 14:160–61.

118. Ikeda, Y. 1968. Gastric brushing cytology under direct-vision. *J. Jap. Soc. Clin. Cytol.* 7:130–31 (in Japanese).

119. Imbriglia, J. E., and Lopusniak, M. S. 1949. Cytologic examination of sediment from esophagus in case of intraepidermal carcinoma of esophagus. *Gastroenterology* 13:457–63.

120. Imbriglia, J. E.; Stein, G. N.; and Lopusniak, M. S. 1951. Cytological study of upper gastrointestinal sediment: Its value as correlated with roentgenologic and clinical findings in diagnosis of cancer. *J.A.M.A.* 147:120–22.

121. Ishioka, K. 1965. Cytological diagnosis of gastric cancer. *J. Jap. Soc. Clin. Cytol.* 4:42 (in Japanese).

122. ———. 1968. Personal communication.

123. Jacobj, W. 1935. Die Zellkerngrosse beim Menschen. *Z. Mikroskopischanat. Forsch.* 38:161–240.

124. Jensen, O., and Schade, R. O. K. 1962. The value of x-chymotrypsin for diagnostic gastric lavage. *Acta Cytol.* 6:475–77.

125. Joekes, T. 1938. Nonsurgical drainage of the gall bladder. *Postgrad. Med. J.* 14:204.

126. Johnson, W. D.; Koss, L. G.; Papanicolaou, G. N.; and Seybolt, J. F. 1955. Cytology of esophageal washings: Evaluation of 364 cases. *Cancer* 8:951–57.

127. Jones, C. M. 1924. The rational use of duodenal drainage: An attempt to establish a conservative estimate of the value of this procedure in the diagnosis of biliary tract pathology. *Arch. Intern. Med.* 34:60.

128. Jones, C. M., and Minot, G. R. 1923. Infectious (catarrhal) jaundice: An attempt to establish a clinical entity; observations on the excretion and retention of the bile pigments and on the blood. *Boston Med. Surg. J.* 189:531.

129. Juniper, K., Jr., and Burson, E. N., Jr. 1957. Biliary tract studies. II. The significance of biliary crystals. *Gastroenterology* 32:60.

130. Kameya, S.; Nakamura, S.; Mizutani, K.; Hayakawa, H.; Higashiyama, S.; and Kutsuna, K. 1964. Gastrofiberscope for biopsy. *Gastroent. Endosc. (Tokyo)* 6:36–40 (in Japanese).

131. Kasugai, T. 1964. Gastric biopsy and cytology by the fibergastroscope. *Gastroent. Endosc. (Tokyo)* 6:187 (in Japanese).

132. ———. 1968. Evaluation of gastric lavage cytology under direct-vision by the fibergastroscope employing Hanks' solution as a washing solution. *Acta Cytol.* 12:345–51.

133. ———. 1968. Gastric lavage cytology and biopsy for early gastric cancer under direct-vision by the fibergastroscope. *Gastroint. Endosc.* 14:205–8.

134. Kasugai, T.; Kato, H.; Ando, A.; Ito, E.; Yagi, M.; Tsubouchi, M.; Yamaoka, Y.; Yoshii, Y.; Hattori, T.; Naito, Y.; Kobayashi, K.; Kobayashi, S.; Koike, A.; and Suchi, T. 1968. A case report of gastric syphilis showing unusual gastroscopic findings. *Stomach Intest. (Tokyo)* 3:315–20.

135. Kidokoro, T.; Soma, S.; Seta, R.; Goto, K.; Yamakara, T.; Taniai, A.; and Katayanagi, T. 1966. Gastric cytology under direct-vision with special reference to suction method (the first report). *Jap. Soc. Clin. Cytol.* 5:31 (in Japanese).

136. Kidokoro, T.; Soma, S.; Seta, R.; Gota, K.; Yamakara, T.; Taniai, A.; Katayanagi, T.; and Asakura, R. 1968. On direct-vision cytology with special reference method. *Stomach Intest. (Tokyo)* 3:1201–10.

137. Klavins, J. V., and Flemma, R. J. 1964. A method for studying the material of the bile ducts. *Acta Cytol.* 8:332–35.

138. Klayman, M. I. 1955. The diagnosis of esophageal carcinoma by exfoliative cytology, including two cases of cardiospasm associated with carcinoma of the esophagus. *Ann. Intern. Med.* 43:33–44.

122

References

139. Klayman, M. I.; Kirsner, J. B.; and Palmer, W. L. 1955. Gastric malignant lymphoma: Increasing accuracy in diagnosis. *Gastroenterology* 29:536–47.
140. Klayman, M. I.; Massey, B. W.; Pleticka, S.; Galambos, J. T.; Brandborg, L.; Kirsner, J. B.; and Palmer, W. L. 1955. Cytological diagnosis of gastric cancer by chymotrypsin lavage. II. Detection of early malignancy. *Gastroenterology* 29: 854–62.
141. Klayman, M. I.; Massey, B. W.; Pleticka, S.; Galambos, J. T.; Brandborg, L.; and Palmer, W. L. 1955. The cytologic diagnosis of gastric cancer by chymotrypsin lavage. I. The accuracy of the method. *Gastroenterology* 29:849–53.
142. Knoerschild, H. E., and Cameron, A. B. 1963. Mucosal smear cytology in the detection of colonic carcinoma. *Acta Cytol.* 7:233–35.
143. Knoerschild, H. E.; Cameron, A. B.; and Zollinger, R. M. 1961. Millepore filtration of colonic washings in malignant lesions of the large bowel. *Amer. J. Surg.* 101:20–22.
144. Kobayashi, S.; Kasugai, T.; Yamaoka, Y.; Yoshii, Y.; and Naito, Y. 1969. Improved technique for gastric cytology utilizing simultaneous lavage and fibergastroscopy. *Gastroint. Endosc.* 15:198–200.
145. Kobayashi, S.; Prolla, J. C.; and Kirsner, J. B. 1970. Brushing cytology of the esophagus and stomach under direct-vision by fiberscopes. *Acta Cytol.* 14:219–23.
146. ———. 1970. Late gastric carcinoma development after previous surgery for benign conditions: Endoscopic and histological studies of the anastomosis and consideration of diagnostic problems. *Amer. J. Dig. Dis.* 15:905–12.
147. ———. 1970. Reactive lymphoreticular hyperplasia of the stomach. *Arch. Int. Med.* 125:1030–35.
148. Kobayashi, S.; Prolla, J. C.; Winans, C. S.; and Kirsner, J. B. 1970. Improved endoscopic diagnosis of gastroesophageal malignancy: Combined use of direct-vision brushing cytology and biopsy. *J.A.M.A.* 212:2086–89.
149. Kobayashi, S.; Prolla, J. C.; Yagi, M.; and Kasugai, T. 1969. Gastroscopic diagnosis of early gastric carcinoma based upon the Japanese classification. *Gastroint. Endosc.* 16:92–97.
150. Kobayashi, S.; Singer, H.; Fagin, R.; Prolla, J. C.; and Kirsner, J. B. 1970. A case of early (superficial) gastric carcinoma. *Stomach Intest. (Tokyo)* 5:365–72.
151. Koss, L. G. 1968. *Diagnostic cytology and its histopathologic bases.* 2d ed. Philadelphia: J. B. Lippincott.
152. Kramer, P. 1950. Symposium on specific methods of treatment: Certain pitfalls in liver function tests. *Med. Clin. N. Amer.* 34:1459.
153. Kurokawa, T.; Saito, T.; Yonemura, H.; Kayaba, M.; Tada, K.; Uruga, K.; Sagara, M.; and Ishioka, K. 1960. Cytological diagnosis of cancer. *Tohoku J. Exp. Med.* 71:209–24.
154. Lagerlof, H. O. 1942. *Pancreatic function and pancreatic disease studied by means of secretin.* New York: Macmillan.
155. Lake, M. 1935. Nonsurgical biliary drainage. *Med. Clin. N. Amer.* 19:677.
156. ———. 1940. The influence of the weight of the duodenal tube tip on its entrance time. *Amer. J. Dig. Dis.* 7:136.
157. ———. 1947. Diagnostic value of the secretin test including a report of nineteen operated or autopsied cases with anatomical studies of the pancreas. *Amer. J. Med.* 3:18.
158. Lecomte, P.; Monges, H.; Legre, M.; Commandre, G.; Giacobre, R.; and Vedel, J. P. 1965. Aspects radiologiques des cancers du moignon gastrique après gastrectomie pour ulcères. *J. Radiol. Electrol.* 46:577.
159. Lemon, H. M. 1951. Clinical value of duodenal drainage in diagnosis of carcinoma of biliary tract and pancreas. *N.Y. J. Med.* 51:2155–58.
160. ———. 1952. The application of cytologic diagnosis to cancers of the stomach, pancreas, and biliary system. *Ann. Intern. Med.* 37:525–33.
161. Lemon, H. M., and Byrnes, W. W. 1949. Cancer of the biliary tract and pancreas: Diagnosis from cytology of duodenal aspiration. *J.A.M.A.* 141: 254–57.
162. Levan, A., and Huschka, T. S. 1959. Nuclear fragmentation: A normal feature of mitotic cycle of lymphosarcoma cells. *Hereditas* 39:137–48.
163. Lippman, C. W. 1914. Simplification of the duodenal tube examination. *J.A.M.A.* 62:911.
164. Loeb, R. A., and Scapier, J. 1951. Rectal washings, technic for cytologic study of rectosigmoid: Preliminary report. *Amer. J. Surg.* 81:298–302.

165. Loeper, M., and Binet, E. 1911. Le cytodiagnostic des affections de l'estomac. *Bull. Soc. Med. Hop.* (*Paris*) 31:563–74.

166. Lopes Cardozo, P. 1954. *Clinical cytology*. Vols. I and II. Leiden: L. Stafleu.

167. Lyon, B. B. V. 1919. Diagnosis and treatment of diseases of the gall bladder and biliary ducts: Preliminary report on a new method. *J.A.M.A.* 73:980.

168. ———. 1923. *Nonsurgical drainage of the gall tract*. Philadelphia: Lea and Febiger.

169. ———. 1937. A plan for the prevention of liver and gallbladder diseases. *Rev. Gastroent.* 4:1.

170. MacDonald, W. C.; Brandborg, L. L., Taniguchi, L.; Beh, J. E.; and Rubin, C. E. 1964. Exfoliative cytological screening for gastric cancer. *Cancer* 17:163–69.

171. MacDonald, W. C.; Brandborg, L. L.; Taniguchi, L.; and Rubin, C. E. 1963. Gastric exfoliative cytology. *Lancet* 2:83–86.

172. ———. 1963. Esophageal exfoliative cytology: A neglected procedure. *Ann. Int. Med.* 59:332–37.

173. MacKenzie, L. L., and Miller, H. B. 1949. Primary carcinoma of the duodenum: Report of a case in which malignant cells were recovered by duodenal drainage. *Gastroenterology* 12:309–11.

174. McNeer, G., and Ewing, J. H. 1949. Exfoliated pancreatic cancer cells in duodenal drainage: Case report. *Cancer* 2:643–45.

175. Marini, G. 1909. Über die Diagnose des Magencarcinomas auf Grund der Cytologischen des Spülwasser. *Arch. Verdaumgskrankh.* 15:251–67.

176. Martinez, I. 1964. Cancer of esophagus in Puerto Rico: Mortality and incidence analysis, 1950–1961. *Cancer* 17:1279–88.

177. Massey, B. W., and Klayman, M. L. 1955. Observations on epithelial cells exfoliated from the upper gastrointestinal tract of patients with pernicious anemia, simple achlorhydria and carcinoma of the esophagus and stomach. *Amer. J. Med.* 230:506–14.

178. Medak, H.; Burkalow, P.; McGrew, E. A.; and Tiecke, R. 1970. The cytology of vesicular conditions affecting the oral mucosa: Pemphigus vulgaris. *Acta Cytol.* 14:11–21.

179. Meltzer, S. J. 1917. The disturbance of the law of contrary innervation as a pathogenetic factor in the diseases of the bile ducts and the gall bladder. *Amer. J. Med. Sci.* 153:469.

180. Merendino, K. A., and Mark, V. H. 1952. An analysis of 100 cases of squamous cell carcinoma of the esophagus. I. With special reference to the delay periods and delay factors in diagnosis and therapy, contrasting state and city and county institutions. *Cancer* 5:52–61.

181. Messelt, O. T. 1960. Results of the cytologic diagnosis of esophageal cancer by smears from material obtained by esophagoscopy; Evaluation of 414 cases. *Acta Un. Int. Cancr.* 16:1364–67.

182. Miles, C. P., and Koss, L. G. 1966. Diagnostic traits of interphase human cancer cells with known chromosome patterns. *Acta Cytol.* 10:21–25.

183. Miller, D. F.; Sikorski, J. J.; Moritz, M. M.; and deLuca, V. A., Jr. 1969. An evaluation of a simplified technique for colonic exfoliative cytology. *Acta Cytol.* 13:53–56.

184. Mlecko, L. M. 1968. Hematemesis associated with "scrape" cytology. *Gastroint. Endoscopy* 15:110–11, 1968.

185. Montgomery, P. W., and von Haam, E. 1951. A study of the exfoliative cytology of oral leukoplakia. *J. Dent. Res.* 30:260–64.

186. Moore, R. D., and Reagan, J. W. 1953. A cellular study of lymph node imprints. *Cancer* 6:606–18.

187. Morson, B. C., and Pang, L. S. C. 1967. Rectal biopsy as an aid to cancer control in ulcerative colitis. *Gut* 8:423–34.

188. Nieburgs, H. E.; Dreiling, D. A.; Rubio, C.; and Reisman, H. 1962. The morphology of cells in duodenal drainage smears: Histologic origin and pathologic significance. *Amer. J. Dig. Dis.* 7:489–505.

189. Nieburgs, H. E.; Werther, J. L.; Hollander, F.; and Janowitz, H. D. 1960. The cytological diagnosis of gastric cancer and evaluation of the abrasive brush technic in 125 cases. *Amer. J. Dig. Dis.* 5:63–72.

190. Niekerk, W. A. van. 1966. Cervical cytological abnormalities caused by folic acid deficiency. *Acta Cytol.* 10:67–73.

191. Nishiura, T., and Tanabe, H. 1968. A case of gastric syphilis. *Stomach Intest.* (*Tokyo*) 3:121–23.

192. Oakland, D. J. 1957. Exfoliative cytology of the colon and rectum. *Brit. Med. J.* 1:1391–94.

References

193. ———. 1961. The diagnosis of carcinoma of the large bowel by exfoliative cytology. *Brit. J. Surg.* 48:353–62.

194. ———. 1962. New way of diagnosis of carcinoma of the large bowel. *Brit. J. Clin. Pract.* 16:707–15.

195. Ohmori, K.; Miwa, T.; and Kumagai, H. 1968. Follow-up studies on healing ulcer in the early carcinoma of the stomach. *Stomach Intest. (Tokyo)* 3:1643–50.

196. Pack, G. T., and Banner, R. L. 1958. The late development of gastric cancer after gastroenterostomy and gastrectomy for peptic ulcer and benign pyloric stenosis. *Surgery* 44:1024–33.

197. Palmer, W. L., and Humphreys, E. M. 1944. Gastric carcinoma: Observations on peptic ulceration and healing. *Gastroenterology* 3:257–74.

198. Panico, F. G. 1952. Improved abrasive balloon for diagnosis of gastric cancer. *J.A.M.A.* 149:1447–49.

199. Panico, F. G.; Papanicolaou, G. N.; and Cooper, W. H. 1950. Abrasive balloon for exfoliation of gastric cancer cells. *J.A.M.A.* 143:1308–11.

200. Papanicolaou, G. N. 1954. *Atlas of exfoliative cytology.* Cambridge, Mass.: Harvard University Press.

201. Papanicolaou, G. N., and Cooper, W. A. 1947. The cytology of the gastric fluid in the diagnosis of carcinoma of the stomach. *J. Nat. Cancer Inst.* 7:357–60.

202. Papanicolaou, G. N., and Traut, H. F. 1941. Diagnostic value of vaginal smears in diagnosis of uterine cancer. *Amer. J. Obstet. Gynec.* 42:193–206.

203. Passarelli, N. M.; Shedd, D. P.; Beres, P.; and Spiro, H. 1963. Exfoliative cytology and early carcinoma of the stomach. *Ann. Surg.* 158:144–47.

204. Peters, H. 1958. Cytologic smears from the mouth: Cellular changes in disease and after radiation. *Amer. J. Clin. Path.* 29:219–25.

205. Petersen, H. 1970. The effect of pure natural secretin on the bicarbonate secretion into the duodenum in man. *Scand. J. Gastroent.* 5:105–11.

206. Prolla, J. C. 1970. On the diagnosis of gastric cancer (comment). *Gastroenterology* 58:124–25.

207. Prolla, J. C.; Kobayashi, S.; and Kirsner, J. B. 1969. Gastric cancer: Some recent improvements in diagnosis based upon the Japanese experience. *Arch. Int. Med.* 124:238–46.

208. ———. 1970. Cytology of malignant lymphomas of the stomach. *Acta Cytol.* 14:291–96.

209. Prolla, J. C.; Kobayashi, S.; Yoshii, Y.; Yamaoka, Y.; and Kasugai, T. 1970. Diagnostic cytology of the stomach in gastric syphilis: Report of two cases. *Acta Cytol.* 14:333–37.

210. Prolla, J. C.; Taebel, D. W.; and Kirsner, J. B. 1965. Current status of exfoliative cytology in diagnoses of malignant neoplasms of the esophagus. *Surg. Gynec. Obstet.* 121:743–52.

211. Prolla, J. C.; Xavier, R. G.; and Kirsner, J. B. 1972. Exfoliative cytology in gastric ulcer: Its role in the differentiation of benign and malignant ulcers. *Gastroenterology.* In press.

212. ———. 1971. Morphology of the exfoliated cells in benign gastric ulcer. *Acta Cytol.* 15:128–32.

213. Prolla, J. C.; Yoshii, Y.; Xavier, R. G.; and Kirsner, J. B. 1971. Further experience with direct-vision brushing cytology of malignant tumors of upper gastrointestinal tract: Histopathologic correlation with biopsy obtained simultaneously. *Acta Cytol.* 15:375–78.

214. Proper, R. 1962. Acridine-Orange fluorescent staining of gastric cytological elements. *Bull. Gastroint. Endosc.* 9:7.

215. Puestow, C. B.; Wurtz, K. G.; and Olander, G. A. 1954. Carcinoma of ampulla of Vater and head of pancreas causing jaundice. *Arch. Surg.* 69:564.

216. Raskin, H. F.; Kirsner, J. B.; and Palmer, W. L. 1958. Exfoliative cytology of the gastrointestinal tract. *Modern trends in gastroenterology,* ed. F. A. Jones, 2:76–91.

217. ———. 1959. Role of exfoliative cytology in the diagnosis of cancer of the digestive tract. *J.A.M.A.* 169:789–91.

218. ———. 1959. Selected practical tests of gastrointestinal function. *Med. Clin. N. Amer.* 43:341–56.

219. Raskin, H. F.; Kirsner, J. B.; Palmer, W. L.; and Pleticka, S. 1964. The clinical value of the negative gastrointestinal exfoliative cytologic examination in cancer suspects. *Gastroenterology* 42:266–74.

220. Raskin, H. F.; Kirsner, J. B.; Palmer, W. L.; Pleticka, S.; and Yarema, W. A. 1958. Gastroin-

testinal cancer: Definitive diagnosis by exfoliative cytology. *Arch. Int. Med.* 101:731–40. *Arch. Surg.* 76:507–16.

221. Raskin, H. F.; Moseley, R. D.; Kirsner, J. B.; and Palmer, W. L. 1961. *Cancer of the pancreas, biliary tract, and liver.* New York: American Cancer Society.

222. Raskin, H. F.; Palmer, W. L.; and Kirsner, J. B. 1959. Exfoliative cytology in diagnosis of cancer of the colon. *Colon Rectum* 2:46–57.

223. Raskin, H. F., and Pleticka, S. 1964. The cytologic diagnosis of cancer of the colon. *Acta Cytol.* 8:131–40.

224. Raskin, H. F.; Wenger, J.; Sklar, M.; Pleticka, S.; and Yarema, W. A. 1958. Diagnosis of cancer of pancreas, biliary tract, and duodenum by combined cytologic and secretory methods. I. Exfoliative cytology and description of rapid method of duodenal intubation. *Gastroenterology* 34:996–1008.

225. Reed, P. I.; Raskin, H. F.; and Graff, P. 1962. Malignant melanoma of the stomach. *J.A.M.A.* 182:178–79.

226. Rehfuss, N., and Nelson, G. M. 1935. *Medical treatment of gallbladder disease.* Philadelphia: W. B. Saunders Co. Chapter 6.

227. Reineboth. 1897. Diagnose des Magencarcinoms aus Spülwasser und Erbrechenen. *Deutsch. Arch. Klin. Med.* 58:62–70.

228. Reinhold, J. B.; Ferguson, L. K.; and Hunsburger, A., Jr. 1937. Composition of human gallbladder bile and its relationship to cholelithiasis. *J. Clin. Invest.* 16:367.

229. Richards, W. C. D., and Spriggs, A. I. 1961. The cytology of gastric mucosa. *J. Clin. Path.* 14:132–39.

230. Richir, C. L., and Lambling, A. 1958. Analyse critique du cytodiagnostic gastrique. *Arch. Mal. Appar. Dig.* 47:1153–62.

231. Roach, J. F.; Sloan, R. D.; and Morgan, R. H. 1952. The detection of gastric carcinoma by photofluorographic methods. III. Findings. *Amer. J. Roentgen.* 67:68–75.

232. Rosen, R. G.; Garret, M.; and Aka, E. 1968. Cytologic diagnosis of pancreatic cancer by ductal aspiration. *Ann. Surg.* 167:427–32.

233. Rosenbach, O. 1882. Über die Anwesenheit von

Geschwulstpartikein in dem durch die Magenpumpe entleeren Mageninhalte bei Carcinoma ventriculi. *Deutsch. Med. Wschr.* 8:452–53.

234. Rosenthal, N., and Traut, H. F. 1951. The mucolytic action of papain for cell concentration in the diagnosis of gastric cancer. *Cancer* 4:147–49.

235. Rossman, M., and Wolf, J. 1956. Accidental gastric biopsies with the Ayre brush. *Gastroenterology* 30:686–89.

236. Rousselot, L. M., and Bauman, L. 1933. Cholesterol crystals and "calcium bilirubinate" granules: Their significance in bile obtained through the duodenal tube. *J.A.M.A.* 100:245.

237. ———. 1933. The diagnostic value of bile obtained through a duodenal tube with special reference to the diagnosis of cholelithiasis. *Ann. Surg.* 98:149.

238. Rubin, C. E. 1952. *Proc. Second National Cancer Conference, Apud* ref. 241.

239. Rubin, C. E. 1955. The diagnosis of gastric malignancy in pernicious anemia. *Gastroenterology* 29:563–87.

240. Rubin, C. E., and Benditt, E. P. 1955. A simplified technique using chymotrypsin lavage for the cytological diagnosis of gastric cancer. *Cancer* 8:1137–41.

241. Rubin, C. E., and Brandborg, L. L. 1969. Gastrointestinal exfoliative cytology. In *Gastroenterologic medicine,* ed. M. Paulson, pp. 331–35. Philadelphia: Lea and Febiger.

242. Rubin, C. E., and Massey, B. W. 1954. Preoperative diagnosis of gastric and duodenal malignant lymphoma by exfoliative cytology. *Cancer* 7:271–88.

243. Rubin, C. E.; Massey, B. W.; Kirsner, J. B.; Palmer, W. L.; and Stonecypher, D. D. 1953. The clinical value of gastrointestinal cytologic diagnosis. *Gastroenterology* 25:119–38.

244. Rubin, C. E., and Nelson, J. F. 1957. Exfoliative cytology as an aid in the differential diagnosis of gastric lesions discovered roentgenologically. *Amer. J. Roentgen.* 77:9–24.

245. Rubin, C. E.; Palmer, W. L.; and Kirsner, J. B. 1952. The present status of exfoliative cytology in the diagnosis of gastrointestinal malignancy. *Gastroenterology* 21:1–11.

246. Rubin, C. E.; Palmer, W. L.; Kirsner, J. B.; Massey, B. W.; and Stonecypher, D. D. 1953.

126

References

Gastrointestinal exfoliative cytology. *Proc. Inst. Med. Chicago* 19:268.

247. Saburi, R.; Ando, T.; Kakihana, M.; Tabayashi, A.; and Yamada, T. 1967. A selective proteolytic lavage method for the cytodiagnosis of early gastric cancer. *Acta Cytol.* 11:473–76.

248. Saito, T.; Yonemura, H.; Kayaba, M.; Tada, K.; Uruga, K.; Sagara, M.; and Ishioka, K. 1960. Fundamental studies on cytological diagnosis of gastric cancer. *Tohoku J. Exp. Med.* 71:237–47.

249. Sandritter, W.; Carl, M.; and Ritter, W. 1966. Cytophotometric measurements of the DNA content of human malignant tumors by means of the Feulgen reaction. *Acta Cytol.* 10:26–30.

250. Schade, R. O. K. 1959. A critical review of gastric cytology. *Acta Cytol.* 3:7–14.

251. ———. 1959. The cytological diagnosis of gastric carcinoma. *Gastroenterologia* 85:190–94, 1956.

252. ———. 1960. *Gastric cytology.* London: Edward Arnold.

253. Schickendantz, G. A. 1963. El citodiagnóstico del cáncer del esófago y del cardias: Análisis de nuestra experiencia. *Prensa Med. Argent.* 50: 2267–75.

254. Segal, H. L.; Friedman, H. A.; and Watson, J. S., Jr. 1948. Problems in diagnosis and treatment in non-calculous gall bladder. *Amer. J. Dig. Dis.* 15: 325.

255. Segi, M., and Kurihara, M. 1966. *Cancer mortality for selected sites in 24 countries. No. 4 (1962–63).* Sendai, Japan: Dept. of Public Health, Tohoku University School of Medicine.

256. Seppala, K. 1961. Exfoliative cytology in gastric malignancy. *Acta Med. Scand.* (Suppl. 363) 169: 1–83.

257. Seybolt, J. F.; Papanicolaou, G. N.; and Cooper, W. A. 1951. Cytology in diagnosis of gastric cancer. *Cancer* 4:286–95.

258. Shay, H., and Riegel, C. 1936. The role of laboratory in the diagnosis of the gallbladder disease. *Amer. J. Med. Sci.* 192:51.

259. Shida, S.; Koike, I.; and Kotaka, H. 1966. The differential diagnosis of gastric tumors by roentgenological, gastroendoscopical, and cytological examinations. In *Proc. First Cong. Internat. Soc. Endoscopy,* pp. 577–85. Tokyo: Hitachi Printing Co.

260. Shida, S., and Tsuda, K. 1966. Cytodiagnosis of gastric malignant lymphoma. *Jap. J. Clin. Med.* 24:1876–88 (in Japanese).

261. Simon, P., and Caussade, L. 1914. Le cytodiagnostic du cancer de l'estomac. *Presse Med.* 22: 265–85.

262. Sinapius, D. 1958. Über das Endothel der Venen. *Z. Zellforsch.* 47:560–630.

263. Smithes, F. 1921. Nonsurgical drainage of the biliary tract: Its usefulness as a diagnosis and therapeutic agent. *Illinois Med. J.* 29:325.

264. Söderström, N. 1966. *Fine-needle aspiration biopsy.* New York: Grune and Stratton.

265. Spjut, H. J.; Margolis, A. A.; and Cook, G. B. 1963. The silicone-foam enema: A source for exfoliative cytologic specimens. *Acta Cytol.* 7:79–84.

266. Staats, O. J.; Robinson, L. H.; and Butterworth, C. E., Jr. 1969. The effect of systemic therapy on nuclear size of oral epithelial cells in folate-related anemias. *Acta Cytol.* 13:84–88.

267. Stout, A. P. 1942. Superficial spreading type of carcinoma of the stomach. *Arch. Surg.* 44:651–57.

268. Stout, A. P. 1953. Tumors of the stomach. In *Atlas of tumor pathology,* sect. 6, fasc. 21. Washington, D.C.: Armed Forces Institute of Pathology.

269. Strandjord, N. M.; Moseley, R. D., Jr.; and Schweinefus, R. L. 1960. Gastric carcinoma accuracy of radiologic diagnosis. *Radiology* 74: 442–51.

270. Sugiura, Y.; Nageta, K.; Ando, S.; Takai, T.; Nishio, S.; Suzuki, T.; Aoki, A.; and Hayashi, K. 1968. A case of gastric tuberculosis. *Stomach Intest. (Tokyo)* 3:769–72.

271. Taebel, D. W.; Prolla, J. C.; and Kirsner, J. B. 1965. Exfoliative cytology in the diagnosis of stomach cancer. *Ann. Int. Med.* 63:1018–26.

272. Takasu, S. 1967. Cytological diagnosis. In *Atlas of early carcinoma of the stomach,* ed. M. Kuru (a cooperative study of the Stomach Cancer Research Staff at the National Cancer Center Hospital, Tokyo). Tokyo: Nakayama-Shoten Co.

273. Takasu, Y., and Takeuchi, T. 1966. Cytodiagnosis of carcinoma of the pancreas. *Jap. J. Clin. Med.* 24: 1889–94 (in Japanese).

274. Terzano, G.; Ramos-Mejia, M. M.; Diaz-Walker, N. G.; Schickendantz, G. A.; and Fagonde, B.

1963. Nuestra experiencia en citologia gástrica. *Prensa Med. Argent.* 50:2339–44.

275. Thabet, R. J., and Knoerschild, H. E. 1960. Millepore filtration technic for colon washings. *Amer. J. Clin. Path.* 34:185–88.

276. Thabet, R. J.; Knoerschild, H. E.; and Hauser, J. L. 1960. Millepore filtration technique for colon washings. *Cytol. Newsletter* 2:2–3.

277. Thabet, R. J., and MacFarlen, E. W. E. 1962. Cytological field patterns and nuclear morphology in the diagnosis of colon pathology. *Acta Cytol.* 6:325–31.

278. Thomson, D. M. P.; Krupey, J.; Freedman, S. O.; and Gold, P. 1969. The radio-immunoassay of circulating carcinoembryonic antigen of the human digestive system. *Proc. Nat. Acad. Sci.* USA 64:161–67.

279. Tobita, Y., and Hara, Y. 1966. Studies on the gastric biopsy and brushings by gastrofiberscope GFB Olympus. In *Proceedings of the First Congress of the International Society of Endoscopy,* pp. 328–29. Tokyo.

280. Tsuneoka, K. 1966. Diagnosis of early gastric cancer with fibergastroscopic biopsy and fibergastroscopic cytology. In *Recent advances in gastroenterology.* Proceedings of the Third World Congress of Gastroenterology, 1:294–99. Tokyo.

281. Turnberg, L. A., and Grahame, G. 1970. Bile salt secretion in cirrhosis of the liver. *Gut* 11:126–33.

282. Umiker, W. O.; Bolt, R. J.; Hoekzema, A. D.; and Pollard, H. M. 1958. Cytology in diagnosis of gastric cancer: Significance of location and pathologic type. *Gastroenterology* 34:859–66.

283. Umiker, W. O.; Pickle, L.; and Waite, B. 1959. Fluorescence microscopy in exfoliative cytology: An evaluation of its application to cancer screening. *Brit. J. Cancer* 13:398–402.

284. Ushigone, S.; Spjut, H. J.; and Noon, G. P. 1967. Extensive dysplasia and carcinoma in situ of esophageal epithelium. *Cancer* 20:1023–29.

285. Ventzke, L. E. 1963. Fluorescence microscopy with Acridine-Orange in gastrointestinal cytology. *Gastroenterology* 45:712–15.

286. Vacca, V. F., and DeLuca, V. A. 1961. A more practical and simplified method of colonic exfoliative cytology: A preliminary report. *Conn. Med.* 30:559–61.

287. Vilardell, F. 1963. *Gastric cytology.* In *Gastroenterology,* 2d ed., ed. H. L. Bockus, 1:771–75. Philadelphia: W. B. Saunders.

288. ———. 1968. Reevaluation of cytologic methods in the diagnosis of malignant lesions of the stomach. In *Progress in gastroenterology,* ed. G. B. J. Glass, 1:129–56. New York: Grune and Stratton.

289. Weiland, D. E.; Kuntz, D. J.; and Childers, D. 1968. Immunologic screening test for carcinoma of the pancreas. *Amer. J. Surg.* 116:700–703.

290. Wenger, J., and Raskin, H. F. 1958. Diagnosis of cancer of pancreas, biliary tract, and duodenum by combined cytologic and secretory methods. II. Secretin test. *Gastroenterology* 34:1009–17.

291. Wied, G. L. 1965. Quality control mechanism for cytology programs (editorial). *Acta Cytol.* 9:407–12.

292. ———. 1968. Computers or cytotechnologists? (editorial). *Acta Cytol.* 12:1–2.

293. Wied, G. L.; Bibbo, M.; Bahr, G. F.; and Bartels, P. H. 1969. Computerized recognition of uterine glandular cells. II. The application of a self-learning program. *Acta Cytol.* 13:662–71.

294. Wigh, R., and Swenson, P.C. 1953. Photofluorography for the detection of unsuspected gastric neoplasms. *Amer. J. Roentgen.* 69:242–67.

295. Wilkinson, S. A. 1948. The value of duodenal drainage: Its place in diagnosis. *Surg. Clin. N. Amer.* 28:587.

296. Williams, D. G.; Truelove, S. C.; Gear, M. W. L.; Massarella, G. R.; and Fitzgerald, N. W. 1968. Gastroscopy with biopsy and cytological sampling under direct-vision. *Brit. Med. J.* 1:535–39.

297. Wisseman, C. L., Jr.; Lemon, H. M.; and Lawrence, K. B. 1949. Cytologic diagnosis of cancer of the descending colon and rectum. *Surg. Gynec. Obstet.* 89:24–30.

298. Witte, S. 1962. Carcinoma ventriculi: Klinik und Cytologie. *Bibl. Gastroent. (Basel)* 5:148–61.

299. ———. 1968. Intravital fluorescent staining with acridine derivates in cytodiagnosis of the upper gastrointestinal tract. *Acta Cytol.* 12:15–17.

300. ———. 1970. Gastroscopic cytology. *Endoscopy* 2:88–93.

301. Witte, S., and Bressel, D. 1965. Die zytologische Diagnose des Ulcus ventriculi. *Deutsch. Med. Wschr.* 90:1100–04.

128

References

302. Yamada, T. 1964. Basic study of the proteolytic enzyme lavage method in the gastric diagnosis, especially in the comparative analysis of the exfoliative tendency of malignant and benign epithelial cells. *Acta Cytol.* 8:19–26.
303. Yamada, T.; Matsumoto, S.; Sankawa, K.; and Seino, Y. 1964. Clinical evaluation of proteolytic enzyme lavage method in the gastric cytodiagnosis: Especially in the detection of early cancer of the stomach. *Acta Cytol.* 8:27–33.
304. Yamagata, S.; Masuda, H.; Oshiba, S.; Ishioka, K.; Ueno, K.; Yamagishi, G.; Mochikusi, F.; Kano, A.; Yago, E.; Yamagata, J.; and Mobiyama, S. 1968. Two cases of early esophagus cancer diagnosed chiefly by esophageal cytology (abstr.). *J. Jap. Soc. Clin. Cytol.* 7:526–27.
305. Yamaoka, Y. 1969. Studies on the lavage cytology of the stomach under direct-vision. *Jap. J. Gastroent.* 66:19–33 (in Japanese).
306. Yoshii, Y.; Takahashi, J.; Yamaoka, Y.; Kasugai, T. 1970. Significance of imprint smear in cytologic diagnosis of malignant tumors of the stomach. *Acta Cytol.* 14:249–53.
307. Ziskin, D. E.; Kamen, P.; and Kittay, L. 1941. Epithelial smears of the oral mucosa. *J. Dent. Res.* 20:386–87.

Index

Handbook and Atlas of Gastrointestinal Exfoliative Cytology